Killing from the Inside Out

"For more than 10 years I have been working with former combatants in different parts of the world, grappling with the profound human cost of their involvement in war/violent political conflict. The dominant discourses of 'post traumatic stress disorder' and 'just war' really do not capture the deep wounding, the soul fragmentation, and inner darkness that many of them continue to be haunted by, especially those who come from religious backgrounds. Meagher's book comes like a much needed breath of fresh air—shining sensitive light on this darkness; pointing with nuanced language to the depth of human wounding in war; highlighting in particular the complicity of the 'just war' tradition in this inner injuring and the difficulties of healing. In this really important book, Meagher combines his own practical wisdom from many years of working with combat veterans with decades of high quality scholarship. As a reflective practitioner I strongly recommend this book to anyone truly interested in transforming the human cost of war."

—WILHELM VERWOERD

International peace and reconciliation worker, Director of Beyond Walls, Cape Town Area, South Africa. His books include: *My Winds of Change* (foreword by Nelson Mandela) and *Journey through Conflict Trail Guide.*

"Professor Meagher has steered us through minefields of thought on just war and justified killing, sacrifice and collateral damage, moral injury and its consequences on individuals and society. His expertise in truth and justice, and extensive experience interviewing individuals and writing about moral injury serve to sharpen our understanding as we help our veterans to wellness. Meagher has written the essential rebuttal to Just War theory. This book should be read by scholars, warriors, clergy, politicians, and anyone caring for those suffering from moral injury related to military service. It is an exceptional tour of Western thought on war and killing, and their justification by our military, religious, and political leaders."

—KIMBERLY MAY, MD

Col (retired), United States Air Force, Medical Corps, currently staff physician, Veterans Administration Medical Center, Leeds, MA.

"The soul of the United States is infected by its addiction to unending war. The suicide rate among soldiers and war veterans has reached epidemic heights. Bob Meagher's seminal and timely work, with its reach from antiquity to today, shows that there never was a just war that would leave its participants unscarred. We live with the terrible consequences of a process from 325 CE when Christian values began to be transposed with imperial values. None of us are hardwired for war, so when we kill each other there will be moral and spiritual injury no matter how justified the war may be."

—REV. MICHAEL LAPSLEY

Founder-Director, Institute for Healing of Memories, Cape Town, South Africa, and author of *Redeeming the Past: My Journey from Freedom Fighter to Healer.*

"Under the skilled hand of this master of the classics, the ancient Greeks cross the eons to bring their wisdom into our time, on issues of vital importance—war and its trail in the souls of killers and their communities. This is the resource for understanding how the religion of the Prince of Peace came to support war. Meagher brings us leaders of the early Christian church, showing us how Christianity came to excuse, if not promote, the industrialized and anonymous killing that war has become. The able professor also weaves in the struggles of current military veterans who struggle for inner peace having done what they were told to do. He manages all this in a manner that gives not despair, but life!"

—AMY BLUMENSHINE

Diaconal Minister, Evangelical Lutheran Church in America, founder of the Coming Home Collaborative, and a co-author of *Welcome Them Home—Help Them Heal*.

"In the field of conflict transformation and peace-building there is a recognized gap between grassroots practitioners who have lived through violent conflict and are working with its legacy, and academics who are considered to be 'experts' while lacking significant on-the-ground experience. Bob Meagher is one scholar who bridges this gulf with integrity, clarity, compassion, and challenge. *Killing from the Inside Out* is a brilliant example of his ability to chart the development of Just War Theory and consider it in the light of the lived experience of human beings sent into battle across the centuries. He doesn't swamp the reader with the vast scope of his personal knowledge but helps us trace easily and engagingly the attitudes to violent conflict and its moral status from the time of the wars of ancient Greece, via the emergence and rise of Christianity during the time of Imperial Rome and forward through the writings of key figures to the present day. He draws fascinating, thought-provoking, and some might say, disturbing parallels between war-making and love-making from a male perspective. He takes seriously the understanding of service personnel deployed as combatants to conflict zones across the world, whose experience illustrates why Just War Theory is dead. I found this book gripping, illuminating, and prophetic. In a so-called civilized world where we continue to accept all too easily the killing of innocents in war, and the sometimes devastating long-term impact on those young people we send into battle to kill on our behalf, it is utterly timely."

—RUTH SCOTT

An Anglican priest, a producer and presenter for the BBC in London, a renowned international peace and conflict resolution worker, and the author of many books, including one on the conflict in Northern Ireland that was made into a feature film starring Liam Neeson.

"Truth often hides, Robert Meagher reminds us, in *Killing from the Inside Out*, especially when the truth challenges our myths, for example, the myth that one can kill another human being and not be damaged by so doing. The truth is no one leaves the battlefield unwounded. Killing wounds the soul. But what if it's a 'just war?' Meagher argues convincingly that to put the adjective 'just' in front of the word 'war' is self-deception."

—JIM FOREST

Co-founded the Catholic Peace Fellowship in 1964 and from 1977 through 1988 was Secretary General of the International Fellowship of Reconciliation. Currently he serves as International Secretary of the Orthodox Peace Fellowship. His books include *The Road to Emmaus: Pilgrimage as a Way of Life, Ladder of the Beatitudes, Praying with Icons, Living With Wisdom: A Biography of Thomas Merton, All Is Grace: A Biography of Dorothy Day,* and *Loving Our Enemies: Reflections on the Hardest Commandment.*

"Bob Meagher lays out a provocative argument: That 'just war,' as a theory and set of principles to guide us in battle, is effectively dead. He tangles with the perverse assumption, passed down through the ages, that there is a just way of taking another person's life, that killing in wartime is somehow different from murder in peacetime. That just war originates in Christian theology, and was invoked in a speech by an American president accepting a Nobel Peace Prize, is even more puzzling. Meagher grapples with not just the collective moral crisis nations go through when they use violence to achieve political ends, but also how ex-soldiers grapple with their own consciences over their actions in the heat of battle, or what he calls 'moral injury.' He comes at the subject not as a pacifist but as an ethicist, marshaling impressive evidence, from the works of St. Augustine to Camus, to make his case. The book recounts the harrowing stories of soldiers who struggle to cope with what they've done in combat, what they've seen, and the scars that stay with them in their postwar lives. Elegantly written and easily accessible to lay readers—his prose unburdened by any military jargon or acronym-soup—*Killing From the Inside Out* is an ideal read for anyone curious about American adventurism abroad, the future of civil-military relations, and the human—and moral—toll of war."

—LIONEL BEEHNER

Founding editor of *Cicero Magazine* and former senior writer at the Council on Foreign Relations.

"Specialists in the field will welcome this book, not only because of its provocative argument, but because there are gems that will enrich even advanced readers's knowledge or thinking. Those who are mostly familiar with international law and secular Just War Theory will find the brisk, sound survey of developments in chapters 4–6 informative; those specializing in the Christian-ethical approach to war will find provocative thoughts in the discussion of Greek literature in chapter 1–3. Even for specialists in Christian ethics or history, the way the author brought out the connections of love and war in Greek literature, and then looked at developments in early Christian thought, should prove stimulating. I am not aware of other works that have explored this so well. I think the book will appeal to people who think about the problem of war from any angle, including philosophical, theological, historical, political, and literary. The book has an accessible style married to serious content that will work well for both beginning and advanced readers. I can see many professors who teach about war and peace—again, from a number of disciplinary angles—procuring the book for their own edification, and then many adopting it for courses. The book will definitely work for both undergraduate and graduate student audiences in any courses that touch on war. The introduction and conclusion and chapters 2 and 3, in particular, are rich with conversation topics. As someone who teaches a basic undergraduate religious-ethics course on war and peace, I would be very interested in assigning this book for the way it puts the charge against Just War Theory so pointedly and for how it could set an ongoing problem for such a course. I can also see courses from philosophy and political-science angles using the book."

—BRIAN STILTNER

Chair of Philosophy, Theology, and Religious Studies, Sacred Heart University, and coauthor of *Faith and Force: A Christian Debate about War.*

"Such Christian thinkers as Augustine and Thomas Aquinas crafted Just War Theory (JWT) in order to limit war. In *Killing from the Inside Out*, Professor Robert Meagher, a poetic writer and brilliant classical scholar, leverages history to provocatively argue that the opposite has actually occurred and JWT has served only to legitimize and inspire war. JWT, he convincingly contends, has also made it tragically easy to deny the existence of moral injury, a condition that commonly afflicts combat veterans and profoundly and negatively affects psyches. How can combat veterans feel guilt or shame, many wonder, if the war they fight is just? Thus the help these afflicted warriors desperately need is withheld from them. Another fundamental truth this bold, beautifully written, and erudite work powerfully conveys is the following: war kills not only those it buries in the ground; it just as surely kills those souls who march home, heads held high while the music plays and their loved ones cheer, yet feeling inside they are forever lost."

—LIEUTENANT COLONEL DOUGLAS A. PRYER

Active-duty counterintelligence officer who has deployed to Kosovo, Afghanistan, and Iraq. He is the author of the book, *The Fight for the High Ground: The U.S. Army and Interrogation During Operation Iraqi Freedom, May 2003–April 2004.*

"*Killing From the Inside Out* examines suicide—the form (of) self-inflicted death resulting within as we acquiesce to war. Robert Emmet Meagher argues persuasively 'just war' is a modern myth, and to kill another is to kill a part of self. This is a thoughtful, timely, and needed book. We need to look war in the eye as our nation, Meagher points out, is on a perpetual warpath. We call it, 'the war against terrorism.' Meagher cites historical thinkers, modern sages, and veterans back from battle. He makes us think and think again as we consider war and its pernicious effect, not only 'out' there, but 'inside' here, inside our singular and collective souls. Read this book. Then ponder it. Then act on it. It just might save a soul—your soul."

—THOMAS C. FOX

As one of the few American correspondents who spoke Vietnamese, Thomas C. Fox covered the war for TIME, *The New York Times* and the *National Catholic Reporter*. He now serves as NCR publisher. His Books include: *Pentecost in Asia: A New Way of Being Church, Sexuality and Catholicism,* and *Iraq: Military Victory, Moral Defeat.*

"Thank you, Professor Meagher, for this honest and courageous precision-guided missile to the heart of just war theory, exposing the institutional and state fear that has inflated and launched this barrage balloon, which over centuries has diverted attention from the truth that there is no such thing as a just war, but just power-hungry greed and insecurity, which lead to just revenge, and worst case for our veterans and others, just suicide. Creation and humanity need us to get out of our comfortable trenches and take this challenge very seriously, to give hope to tortured minds, hearts, and souls, and help us all find just peace."

—REV. ANDREW RAWDING

Graduate of the Royal Military Academy Sandhurst, former combat infantry officer in South Armagh, Northern Ireland and, after ordination to the priesthood, Royal Marine chaplain, who served with Royal Marines and U.S. Marines in Afghanistan

"For millennia, young men (and increasingly women) have been told that war is a place in which they will win glory and honor. When soldiers write about their battlefield experiences, however, one notices a fundamental disconnect between their perspective and the way in which war is popularly conceived. By and large, soldiers discover on their own that little is gained in war and all too much is lost. It is no long stretch, then, to indict the intellectual tradition of just war in this cultural dissonance, that the moral pain suffered post-combat is in part inflicted by communities and voices who do not know the true nature of war.

Just war was initially a pastoral response to the problem of martial pain by a North African bishop who fielded conflicted correspondence from the highest ranking of soldiers. Instead of turning to three centuries of church history built upon the experience of soldier saints and military martyrs, Augustine turned to a pagan jurist. Just war as a theological project was doomed from the start, and Meagher provides here for us its two thousand year long obituary.

Not all have given up hope that the tradition may have something to positively contribute to the actual well being of soldiers, as Augustine's pastoral instincts should be commended. It cannot be denied, however, that, though Meagher's criticisms of the just war tradition cut to the core, they are sorely needed. One need not agree with him that it be torn up from its roots to be profoundly challenged by his work here. His writing wonderfully balances scholarly research with literary tact and will be appreciated by academic and popular audiences alike."

—LOGAN MEHL-LAITURI

candidate, M.Litt Scripture & Theology, St. Andrews, Fife, UK

"Meagher's book, *Killing From the Inside Out*, resonates deeply with my own experience of war in Iraq, and with the emotional distress I felt in its wake. His account of the dark history of 'Just War' theory is a brilliant and lucid explanation of how that doctrine has been used since its creation, not as an earnest attempt to distinguish just from unjust wars, but as a discursive device used to manipulate public opinion and martial support for Christian-based war narratives. The ugly catch, that Meagher has so forcefully demonstrated for us, is that with 'Just War' doctrine as the basis for our wars, and with the 'good against evil' rationale for fighting, there comes a moral apocalypse in the aftermath for the veterans who have done the fighting and who, upon coming home, are left with no cultural or social means for contending with the horrors they've witnessed and the violence they've taken part in, all at the behest of a largely indifferent nation. *Killing From the Inside Out* is an urgent message for all the populations of Western society; America is not the first nation to invoke 'Just War' doctrine to propel its violent policies and it surely won't be the last. Let this book serve as the means by which we resist such morally dubious claims for war."

—TYLER BOUDREAU

served twelve years in the Marine Corps infantry, deployed to Iraq in 2004, and is the author of *Packing Inferno: The Unmaking of a Marine*

"There is a logical tension in the twin ideas that killing is immoral and war is necessary. Professor Meagher has diligently traced the logical, theological, and political arguments that have shaped this debate in Western societies for the past two thousand years. His book has never been more relevant than in our era where advanced weaponry has made too many people heedless of the costs of battle. I hope that his work illuminates for us that in the world of perpetual conflict we have created, it may be time to restore order."

—TIMOTHY KUDO

a former U.S. Marine infantry officer who served tours in Iraq and Afghanistan

Killing from the Inside Out

Moral Injury and Just War

Robert Emmet Meagher

Foreword by
Stanley Hauerwas

Afterword by
Jonathan Shay

CASCADE *Books* · Eugene, Oregon

Cascade Books
An Imprint of Wipf and Stock Publishers
199 W. 8th Ave., Suite 3
Eugene, OR 97401

www.wipfandstock.com

ISBN 13: 978-1-62564-692-7

Cataloguing-in-Publication data:

Meagher, Robert E.

    Killing from the inside out : moral injury and just war / Robert Emmet Meagher ; foreword by Stanley Hauerwas ; afterword by Jonathan Shay.

    xxii + 162 pp. ; 23 cm. Includes bibliographical references and index.

    ISBN 13: 978-1-62564-692-7

    1. War neuroses. 2. War—Moral and ethical aspects. 3. Veterans—Mental health—United States. 4. Post-traumatic stress disorder. 5. War—Psychological aspects. 6. Just war doctrine. I. Hauerwas, Stanley, 1940–. II. Shay, Jonathan. III. Title.

RC550 .M43 2014

Manufactured in the U.S.A.

For my grandchildren, Noah and Lucy

They

The Bishop tells us: "When the boys come back
They will not be the same; for they'll have fought
In a just cause: they lead the last attack
On Anti-Christ; their comrade's blood has bought
New right to breed an honorable race.
They have challenged Death and dared him face to face."
"We're none of us the same!" the boys reply.
"For George lost both his legs; and Bill's stone blind;
Poor Jim's shot through the lungs and like to die;
And Bert's gone syphilitic: you'll not find
A chap who's served that hasn't found *some* change."
And the Bishop said: "The ways of God are strange!"

—SIEGFRIED SASSOON

Contents

Foreword

BOB MEAGHER AND I were colleagues in the Department of Theology at the University of Notre Dame for a number of years beginning in 1970. I quite frankly did not know what to make of Meagher. He had been a Notre Dame undergraduate who, like many at that time, had been deeply influenced by Father John Dunne, CSC. Father Dunne, who recently died, was a legend on the campus of Notre Dame. Students poured into his courses because he was a person of great insight drawing on the literatures of the world to illumine what it means to be a human being. Meagher followed in Dunne's path, developing a way to think about our lives in a manner that challenged the disciplinary boundaries that make up the modern university. At the time I was a much more conventional thinker—thus my problem of not knowing what to make of Meagher.

Meagher left Notre Dame to teach at Hampshire College. That school seemed to be a perfect fit for Meagher because Hampshire was a school built on the presumption that if undergraduates were to get the education they needed to face the realities of our time the disciplinary divisions must be challenged. Because of his move to Hampshire, however, Meagher and I simply lost touch with one another—at least we lost touch until Meagher sent me this extraordinary book. I had no idea that he had spent so much time and scholarly attention on thinking through the moral challenges war entails.

So it is a great pleasure and honor that he has asked me to write the Foreword to his book. To be asked to write the Foreword not only reconnects us after years of not being in touch, but it also suggests over those same years we have come to share judgments I suspect we would not have anticipated when we were colleagues at Notre Dame. I do not mean to suggest we agree about the morality or, if you prefer, the immorality of war, but I think the reader of this book who knows something of my account of war will find some deep continuities between Meagher and me.

In truth, Meagher's work on war continues to represent the kind of difference I suggested above characterized our intellectual differences when we were colleagues at Notre Dame. That is to say, Meagher continues to have a scholarly control of literatures I simply cannot pretend to know well. Thus one of the characteristics of this book is its ability to show how the way war is depicted in the literatures of Greece informs our current understanding of war. I can only admire his ability to utilize literatures that are normally not part of the discussions about the morality of war.

Those literatures, moreover, are quite important for the development of one of his major themes in this book. Without in any way trying to undercut the use of just war as a way to evaluate the morality of war, Meagher has directed our attention to what war does to combatatants in order to help us better understand why war is such a problematic enterprise. Meagher takes no prisoners, but that does not mean his account of what participation in war does to soldiers is not extremely important. Drawing on literatures of many cultures, Meagher helps us see how the very imaginative possibility that I may have to kill someone constitutes a challenge to our everyday morality that is not easily integrated into an ongoing way of life.

I need to make sure there is no misunderstanding about what I have just written. I do not mean to suggest to the reader that Meagher has failed to provide an account of the development of just war theory. The exact opposite is the case, as he has given us a tour of the development of just war theory that will be of great use for those who find just war reflection crucial for any attempt to better understand the morality of warfare. His account of the relation of the church's development of an ethics of sex and just war alone is worth the price of the book. His account of the role of Ambrose in the development of just war reflection is a genuine contribution to our knowledge that, as far as I know, no one has developed with the depth he has.

I am convinced his emphasis on what war does to combatants is a decisive intervention that helps us better understand the morality of war. As a person committed to Christian nonviolence, I fear that many assume a commitment to nonviolence carries with it a negative judgment against those who participate in war. Meagher challenges that presumption by helping us see that those who dissent from war and those who have participated in war share more in common than the stereotype of either would suggest. That war wounds us morally is not only true of those who prosecute the violence of war; it is true of all whom war touches.

Toward the end of this book Meagher quotes Camus to the effect that the years they have gone through, referring to the years of interwar Europe, "have killed something in us." Drawing on a wide range of literature, Meagher helps us, warrior and pacifist alike, to discover what war has done to us. He concludes his book with the strong claim that just war theory has been a cover for the support of war without in any decisive way limiting the violence of war. That is a challenge that hopefully those committed to just war will take seriously.

I began by locating my early relationship to Meagher, noting at the time I was not quite sure what to make of him as a person or a thinker. I am not sure our reconnecting after so many years means I now have a better grasp of the character of his intelligence. But I do know one thing: he possesses a courage that enables him to challenge the myths that surround war with a bracing honesty that is as powerful as it is unusual. I sincerely hope this book will find a wide readership.

Stanley Hauerwas

Author of *War and the American Difference:
Theological Reflections on Violence and National Identity*;
Gilbert T. Rowe Professor Emeritus of Divinity and Law,
Duke University

Preface

"WHAT I'VE TRIED TO do, very frankly," asserted Secretary of Defense Leon Panetta testifying at a joint hearing of the House Armed Services and Veterans Affairs committees in late September 2012, "is to make sure that . . . all of the military leadership kick ass on this issue."[1] The "issue" preying on him was not the defeat of the Taliban or the extermination of al-Qaeda, much less contingency planning for feared budget cuts. No, the issue Panetta had in mind and labeled a "top Pentagon priority" was the runaway suicide rate in the military, averaging thirty-three suicides per month in 2012, roughly one every seventeen hours. Even this number—representing confirmed suicides among active-duty troops—falls far short of the dark truth. Off the Department of Defense's map and spreadsheets are the veterans who, weeks or months or years after their war service, take their lives, often without much national or even local notice. Here the numbers are even more shocking—twenty-two a day in February 2013, nearly one every hour. Then there are the uncounted other deaths among veterans that result from clearly self-destructive behavior, but for a range of reasons are either not seen or reported as suicides. And what of the broken survivors, the legions of others whose lives, though spared in combat, have sprung so many leaks that they spend the rest of their days and nights just staying afloat?

While we were meant to be reassured and hopeful in the news that our Defense Secretary and the military leadership was "on this," we were and are entitled to doubt that this is a crisis that can be resolved by "kicking ass," which the Pentagon admittedly knows how to do. The reality is that the

1. Zoroya, "Military Leaders," 1.

military and the Veterans Administration, in particular, have been aware of this crisis for decades, ever since Vietnam, with little result. For all their doubtlessly sincere concern, the military elite appear at a loss to stanch the flow of self-shed blood in their ranks. They speak of the enormous stress of multiple deployments, the rising incidence of PTSD (post-traumatic stress disorder), and the hidden torments of traumatic brain injury. These are the categories of generals and staff clinicians, concerned above all to maintain troop strength and battle-readiness. To begin to grasp the crisis at hand they need instead to take their eyes off the numbers and to look instead straight into the eyes of one man or woman at a time, someone far below them in rank, someone who has not yet gone dark in death but is daily going dark in life. Even more they need to listen for hours, days, even years—as long as it takes—until they understand what is going so terribly wrong.

Our military, any military, knows all about killing the enemy. It is what they do, and our forces do it more effectively than most. What we are painfully coming to realize, however, is that we are also especially good at killing our own, killing them "from the inside out," silently, invisibly. This is the way the mother of Noah Pierce explained what the army and the war did to her son so that he could imagine nothing better to do with his life than to end it. What brought Noah, a veteran of two deployments in Iraq, to this point was no mystery to his mother. It was an atrocity. The military knows all about body count, but neither understands nor acknowledges "soul count." Kicking ass will get us nowhere as a nation. Searching our soul is more to the point, and this is what this book sets out to do.

Killing from the Inside Out is the work of years—years of reading and years of listening—nearly fifty years, in fact, of research, teaching, activism, and advocacy. It is a profoundly personal work for me, because war invaded my life and family many years ago and, like an army of occupation, has never truly left. I find no fascination in war, only grief and responsibility. For most of my seventy years I have been aware of its wreckage, especially human wreckage, and have wanted to play some small part in closing and healing the wounds it inflicts, especially those wounds inflicted so deeply that they can hide even as they kill. From the start it has been a search for understanding, because without it we are useless, just as I am convinced the military is useless or worse in their mostly blind and misdirected efforts to address the suicide epidemic in their ranks. Above all else I resolved to listen, long and hard, and with an open mind and heart, to how veterans describe and self-diagnose their inner pain, darkness, and desolation, trusting that they know best their own condition. To my surprise, in all this, I have found that on many occasions my tentative responses—drawn from my own scholarship and experience—to others' experiences and stories proved revealing and helpful; so we passed together from monologue to dialogue, from narrative to discussion. And, at first imperceptibly, this book was conceived.

The actual birth of my project occurred during a particular conversation several years ago with a close friend, an ex-Marine captain who served in Iraq and took part in the invasion of Fallujah. He talked and I listened as he argued that any serious critique of war—past, present, or future—was and is and will be undermined before it starts by the unthinking and all but universal acceptance of just war doctrine. He went on to say that the just war theory has to be taken down, discredited, revealed for the lie that it is, and, he added, looking at me, "You're the one to do it." This was a challenge that I could not easily dismiss. So I went to work.

Why would a Marine officer and combat veteran, we might ask, put out a "hit" on the just war theory? What is this "theory" anyway and why does it matter so much? The deceptive and destructive core of the Christian just war doctrine can be stated very simply. It is the claim that wars, or at least some wars, and all the killing and destruction they entail, are—in addition to being necessary—good and right, even virtuous and meritorious, pleasing in the sight of God. This calls for a new species or category of homicide: "killing" that is radically distinct from "murder," a distinction that hadn't previously existed in Christian ethics. "Murder" violates the will of God and darkens the soul of the murderer, but the other, "new" kind of killing doesn't. The difference lies not in the level of violence, death, suffering, and destruction involved but in the "intention" of the killer. If the intention is to do the will of God, which the tradition identifies as the will of the church and its ordained spokesmen or else the will of a legitimate secular sovereign authority, and if all that is done is done with "love," or at least not in hate, then there can be no moral injury because there has been no moral infraction, no sin. If the intention is pure, all is well in heaven and so on earth.

The origin of this foundational claim lay not in the New Testament, nor in early Christian theology and practice, but rather in a practical necessity and political convenience. Once the Christian church found itself in a position of power, which is to say that once the Roman Empire became the Holy Roman Empire, the exercise of lethal force and the waging of war, that is, killing, became its ecclesiastical responsibility. In fact, service in the army, the imperial legions, was confined to baptized Christians. How, then, could the Christian church say that military service was sinful? How could it maintain and deploy an army of Christians whose very service put their souls at peril? A pacifist church was one thing, but a pacifist Christian empire was something very different, and untenable. Augustine, and his mentor Ambrose, both of whom had once aspired to a secular career in the imperial service, came up with the solution, a new theory of war and killing that would not only permit but endorse killing for "God and Country," as it were. It was from the beginning a doctrine of convenience—conceived, promulgated, and perpetuated by men who themselves, as clerics, men of God, would personally eschew service in the military and the conduct of war. They and their successors in the tradition would readily raise a hand to bless the troops but never themselves lift a hand to wield a sword. There would be no blood on their hands. War and killing, now blessed, soon became not the lesser of two evils but a positive good.

Invented in a theological lab, just war and virtuous killing, as soon as they were tested in the field, proved useful for some and devastating to others. The "others" were the combatants, the killers and their victims. The shocking truth was that the "side effects" of just war on these unordained others were of little concern. Not even civilian casualties, however massive, were finally allowed to question its efficacy. Church and state were not about to condemn war, any more than they are today, not at least *their* wars; so war had to be good. Or rather, "our" wars had to be good, and those who serve in them do no wrong, ever, so long as they serve the cause and follow orders. Every war is just, from the perspective of those waging it, and every killer is a hero, to the side they are on. That is the wall our veterans still run up against today. They are expected to deny their own pain, ignore what war has taught them, and take up their civil status as heroes. The rest is supposedly "in their heads," or more precisely in their brains, and there are on offer perfectly good drugs to deal with that. From the beginning of the just war tradition, the powers-that-be needed their wars, and so they created their heroes. Nothing about that has changed, including the confusion and resentment of the returning warrior at the reception he comes home to. It "baffle[s] him," writes Kevin Powers, an Iraq war veteran and author of the acclaimed novel *The Yellow Birds*, "because he immediately remembers what he has actually done, the acts of violence he's committed for which he's being thanked, and it just doesn't make sense. And he doesn't get to hide from the fact that he must account for what he's done."[2] The truth is that just war theory has never made sense to those with blood on their hands nor to those whose blood it was. But their voices have mattered little and could be ignored until now.

The reason, then, why just war doctrine lies at the root of our complacency with war as well as our inability to comprehend the fact of our military "heroes" marching off to take their own lives is that so long as we cling to the moral justification of our wars we remain blind to the moral injury they inflict. Taking on the millennia-old tradition of just war, however, is no slight task. We are, after all, attached to it, invested in it as a nation. It is a lie that has deep and deeply revered roots, particularly in Christian belief, and must be torn up by those roots rather than felled with a single whack.

Uprooting an elaborate, longstanding lie, told and retold across millennia, demands a journey back into time. "If you don't know history, you don't know anything. You're a leaf that doesn't know it's part of a tree."[3] Today's stories of suicide and moral injury are only the latest expression of a much older story. Their rarely examined roots reach deep into the history of war and its consequences. If we don't know how the stories we live and tell today are connected to the story of the past, we don't know anything. In the words of Goethe, "If anyone is unable to give an account of three thousand years of human history, he lives in darkness, inexperienced. He lives from day to day."[4] When each new day brings another veteran suicide, we can no longer afford to live from day to day, confused and uncomprehending.

This book, from cover to cover, is a conversation across time, as it must be, because the understanding sought and shared here does not finally belong to any one time, any more than do war and the profound moral injury it inflicts on all who wage it. It is all about listening to stories—some from today and some from the past—because the present is never without roots and the past is never really past. Military suicide today is not some undecipherable, modern or even postmodern, aberration, without deep roots in our shared human past. Rather, it is the lamentable legacy of a long tradition of justified war and inevitable moral injury.

As it is mostly used today, the term "moral injury" designates the violation, by oneself or another, of a personally embedded moral code or

2. Williams, "Writing Differently," 3.

3. These words are widely attributed to Michael Crichton, but I have never seen them traced to a specific source in his writings.

4. Cited in Jonas, "Change and Permanence," 526. The translation here is mine.

value resulting in deep injury to the psyche or soul. It is what used to be called sin. The haunting question raised and pursued relentlessly in this book is "how can there be moral injury in a just war?" The traditional and mostly unquestioned answer is that there can't be. The idea that dutiful service to one's country in a just war can be simply "wrong," putting at risk one's humanity and very soul, is blasphemous and unthinkable to nearly everyone except those who have experienced it to be the case. It is an idea that many or most veterans are unwilling to express, for they know the anger and resentment they will provoke with their words. Timothy Kudo, a Marine captain who served in both Iraq and Afghanistan, learned this when he submitted a piece to the *Washington Post*, in January 2013, titled "I Killed People in Afghanistan. Was I Right or Wrong?" This was a question that on his own admission he never examined or resolved until his return home. "We were simply too busy," he explained, "to worry about the morality of what we were doing."[5] Now, however, he thinks about it every day, because he knows and lives with the "ethical damage" that killing does to the killer, which he admits "may be worse than the physical injuries we sustain."[6] The best he can do is to say that "killing is always wrong, but in war it is necessary."

As was soon made vociferously clear, Timothy Kudo's "best" was not good enough for some armchair patriots back home, who support the troops, welcome them home, and don't want to hear what they have done or learned. Thanks for your service, but no thanks for your comments. Perhaps understandably, Kudo's brief, honest, and heart-wrenching admission that the killing he did for his country was wrong—not because the war was unjust but because killing is always wrong—spawned a storm of outrage and dismissal. One particularly offensive response to Kudo was an article that soon appeared in the *National Review*, entitled "A Morally Confused Marine," in which the author said that he has "to wonder why, given his belief that killing is always wrong, Timothy Kudo ever enlisted in the Marines."[7] The fact is that when Kudo enlisted the morality of killing was not on his mind. It was a question he hadn't yet asked. It was the experience and inner aftermath of killing that raised the question and brought him to where he is now. He learned from doing, rather than from reading. The fact

5. Kudo, "I Killed People," 1.

6. Ibid., 2.

7. Prager, "Morally Confused," 2.

is that Captain Kudo, far from succumbing to moral confusion, has come to moral clarity, the moral clarity that is the core aspiration of this book.

Timothy Kudo is not alone in his clarity. The telling truth is that a great many combat veterans, having followed all the rules, are haunted more by what they have done than by what they have endured in war. Those who work with veterans to help heal their inner, invisible wounds know that the deepest and most intractable PTSD has its roots in what veterans perceive as the evil they have done and been a part of. They all too often see themselves as criminals, not because they have committed war crimes but because they have become convinced by their own experience of the essential criminality of war. Needless to say this is a conviction that neither the military nor the government is prepared to hear and take seriously. "Kicking ass" does not include facing the possibility that all killing kills something in the killer and that, as a result, there is no such thing as killing without dying, a false promise that has defined the strategy and propaganda of Western war-makers ever since Alexander mesmerized the world with his winner-take-all conquests. The untold stories of those conquests belong to his warriors and their victims, who know that killing is all about dying, even for those who walk away from war seemingly alive and unscathed.

Timothy Kudo, make no mistake, is not a pacifist. He was in his *Post* piece and has been in his many subsequent responses and interviews unmistakably clear that he believes that killing is necessary in war. Necessary—not the same as honorable, praiseworthy, or even right. He has made equally clear that he remains a Marine, that he is prepared to do his duty, follow the orders given him, and that he is proud of his service to the Corps and his country. What makes him different from his unthinking, or should we say confused, critics is that he knows and bears the cost of that service. He knows what killing has done and will do to him. "War makes us killers," he writes. "We must confront this horror directly if we're honest about the true costs of war. . . . I'm no longer the 'good' person I once thought I was. There's nothing that can change that; it's impossible to forget what happened, and the only people who can forgive me are dead."[8] Timothy Kudo is thankfully one of the survivors. Countless others, like Noah Pierce, who have expressed or thought these same words, are gone. All the more reason for listening to Kudo and to other wounded prophets like him, instead of dismissing him, as Dennis Prager did, saying that Kudo's "moral compass"

8. Kudo, "I Killed People," 2.

was broken and in need of recalibration, that is, in need of being put in sync with just war doctrine.

Since the time of Constantine, the first Christian emperor, and of Augustine, the first theologian to develop a Christian defense of war, just war doctrine has served to license and legitimize state and ecclesiastical violence and to draw a convenient, if imaginary, line between killing and murder. It has come to be assumed that the Bible tells us so, and Augustine never tired of reminding us of this. The Bible, however, says no such thing. The fact that the Bible, in Exodus, uses more than one word for killing is true, but it is equally true that it uses them interchangeably. Augustine didn't read Hebrew, and he knew less Greek than most of my beginning students. What he did know was what he wanted the Bible to say, about how murder is one thing and killing is another, and how God's commandments prohibit the one and not the other. And that was enough for his purpose, which was to justify killing, as well as less-than-lethal uses of violence, including torture. Yes, it was not John Yoo who first justified torture in the United States. Augustine beat him to it by sixteen centuries, at least for adherents to just war doctrine, a vast cohort including nearly everyone today. The lone dissenters—mostly veterans and members of various "peace churches" such as the Quakers, Mennonites, Amish, and Church of the Brethren—together make up perhaps 1 percent of us.

After each of the "great wars" of the twentieth century, when the nations of the world entertained the possibility of a world without war and came together to try to make that happen, promising to outlaw war once and for all, it was the doctrine of just war, the birthright and bequest of the Catholic Church, long since discredited and discarded by international lawyers and the family of nations, that was revived and reenlisted in the nick of time to drape in some "legitimacy" the American wars of the last five decades in Vietnam, Afghanistan, and Iraq, as well as the less easily designated endless war on terror. While we may wonder how much this legitimacy is really worth, it was enough for President Barack Obama to feel secure in invoking the just war theory in his, of all things, Nobel Peace Prize acceptance speech and in defending his targeted assassinations in Pakistan and elsewhere, by reassuring a skeptical world and American citizenry that he studies and follows to the letter the just war teachings of Augustine and Aquinas. How is it in that case, we might ask, that the drone pilots in his just war, who do their fighting and killing in the risk-free, climate-controlled security of their cubicles in Nevada and northern Virginia, suffer the same or worse levels of trauma, guilt, and shame as their more front-line comrades in Helmand Province? This is but one strand in our story, and but one of the questions and contradictions I set out to examine and unravel in the central narrative and argument of this book.

The aim of this book is, then, to pull up, from its roots, the just war tradition, to reveal its deadly legacy, and to point to a future beyond just war. To move beyond just war, however, is not the same as moving beyond war. Two eminent men of conscience in the twentieth century—Dietrich Bonhoeffer and Albert Camus, one a Christian theologian and the other an avowed agnostic—were convinced of this. Both refused to distinguish between killing and murder and to justify killing. Yet both, in the face of the evil that was the Third Reich, advocated and embraced the sword, Camus in the Resistance and Bonhoeffer in the effort to assassinate Hitler. Neither man was morally confused, or for that matter morally innocent. They knew that killing is always wrong but accepted quite grudgingly that it is sometimes—in dark times—necessary, as the lesser of two evils. Moving beyond just war, in the first place, means renouncing any effort to justify the war one wages and to accept, therefore, the moral consequences, the moral injury, of such engagement. Then, in that place of despondent darkness, there will one day come the renunciation of all war. Otherwise, as has been realized, perhaps for the first time, by my generation, the children of Oppenheimer, we are all lost.

For this reason, among many, I look to our nation's combat veterans for the prophetic vision, courage, and conviction that will be needed for us to take the first steps beyond war and to undertake the novel challenge of establishing and maintaining peace without arms, without killing. Augustine once wrote that without darkness we cannot know or relish light, and without evil we won't know or love the good. Vietnam veterans had their own way of putting this with respect to their experience of darkness and evil: "If you didn't go, you don't know." But they, like today's veterans, do know, in their bones, in their souls, that every war should be our last, no matter the cost. And we need to listen to and learn from them, which is ultimately what I have tried to do in writing this book.

Therefore I begin my thanks with all of the many veterans of war and conflict who have in their spoken and written words tried to teach us what we need to know. I regret, and at the same time am thankful, that these teachers are too numerous for me to count, much less to name here. To acknowledge these debts would be a book in itself, and even then I would inevitably leave someone out. Better to acknowledge more simply that my work is born of reading and, even more, of listening, and I just hope I have been faithful to all of the pain, wisdom, and trust that have been shared with me in those exchanges. Lastly, in dedicating this book to my grandchildren, Noah and Lucy, I have in mind all the world's children with whom they will live and grow old, sharing a planet ever smaller, more precious, and more imperiled. May they all together, hand in hand, embrace peace and pass it on, along with life, to their children.

1

Introduction

Moral Injury Then and Now

T HAT WE LIVE TODAY in an age of endless war is a mantra intoned
so often as to keep an easily distracted nation ever-mindful that it
needs to be vigilant, even preemptive, and above all aggressively armed.
War has become our natural posture, our national default position, and
we are more or less comfortable with it and its consequences. After all,
our lives go on as we feel they should without grave risk or injury, provided we belong to the 99 percent who never see the face of war up front.
That honor, as we like to think of it, belongs to our men and women in
arms, our heroes, whom we thank for their service and for whom we tie
yellow ribbons and all too often lower our flags halfway.

It is a more careless than truly grateful nation, however, that watches
and applauds its sons and daughters as they go off to war and return, and
yet fails to notice or care for long that they come back different and often
desperate. The fact that the majority of their wounds are invisible is no
excuse. What we cannot see we can still come to know through listening.

Fortunately, not all combat veterans return from war with wounds to
their bodies or to their souls. But many do, too many. Those who come back
without limbs or eyes, those who will never work or even walk again, often
or maybe even most of the time receive the care they deserve; but those
who come back without a scar—silent, hollowed out, shadowed, and overlooked until they take their agony out on themselves or others—rarely find

1

recognition, much less healing. Yet what would healing mean for them? For the most part, we as a nation haven't a clue, and there are reasons for that. One of the central tasks of this book will be to examine the reasons why the moral torment of so many veterans mostly falls on deaf ears.

It may be that the question simply makes no sense to those who have thought little and experienced even less of war. How, for example, can those who have served their country, risked death and injury, observed the rules of war, and followed orders—in what the president of the United States, Barack Obama, in his 2009 Nobel Peace Prize acceptance speech labeled a morally justified use of violence—be in need of spiritual healing or "repentance"? Repentance for what? The clergy, and their congregations with them, regardless of faith or denomination,[1] rarely perceive the possibility of sin in national service. Most of them long ago accepted one or other version of the traditional just war theory, regularly revised and recalibrated across the centuries to certify the moral legitimacy of lethal violence, provided certain conditions are met. Meeting those conditions is, most everyone assumes, the responsibility of the White House and the Pentagon, not that of individual citizens who need to take their government at its word. In general, pastors on the home front, like chaplains in the combat zone, support the troops, as they should, as well as everything the troops are commanded to do, which they arguably should not. The truth is that a great many combat veterans, having followed all the rules, are haunted more by what they have done than by what they have endured in war. Those who work with veterans to help heal their inner, invisible wounds know that the deepest and most intractable PTSD (post-traumatic stress disorder) has its roots in what veterans perceive as the evil they have done and been a part of. They all too often see themselves as criminals, not because they have committed war crimes but because they have become convinced by their own experience of the essential criminality of war. Needless to say this is a conviction that neither the military nor the government is prepared to hear and take seriously.

To whom, then, if not to the clergy, can the morally injured, spiritually desolate veteran turn? The ranks of secular caregivers attending to those suffering from invisible wounds are filled by therapists and counselors with one or other cluster of qualifying letters after their names—psychiatrists,

---

1. As I have already stated in the Preface, those denominations known as the "peace churches"—Quakers, Mennonites, Amish, Church of the Brethren—are clear exceptions to this generalization, as are many American Buddhists; and all of these combined represent far less than 1 percent of the U.S. population, as do the military.

clinical psychologists, and social workers and psychiatric mental health nurses. Armed with the latest edition of the DSM, *The Diagnostic and Statistical Manual of Mental Disorders,* and informed by the vast clinical literature addressing battle trauma, what they see in and hear from their patients more often than not looks like and sounds like classic, standard, well-documented PTSD (post-traumatic stress disorder) or TBI (traumatic brain injury), and they proceed accordingly in weighing their treatment options. Some of these caregivers, however, especially those who have listened longer and more openly to their patients, have begun to question whether they truly grasp the source and extent or even the nature of their patients' suffering. When combat veterans speak to them of the impenetrable darkness in which they now live out their days, much less their nights, or try to convey the shame and guilt that consumes them, psychiatrists may well and often do question whether the most appropriate solution is to whip out their Rx pads. When veterans, even those not previously or particularly religious, report that their souls are dead or that they have lost their humanity and want it back, many MDs and PhDs on the frontlines of veteran care rightly wonder why they are the ones to be hearing this. But if not they, then who? With no ready answer to this question at hand, they do their best, often generously overstepping their professional training and/ or personal beliefs and disbeliefs to acknowledge the obvious suffering of others and to just be there to listen.

The inner damage and pain that even the most qualified and concerned caregivers hesitate to address is what many today diagnose as "moral injury."[2] Moral injury is not a new concept, much less a new reality, as will become painfully clear in the course of this book. All that is relatively recent is the term "moral injury," freshly minted in the minds of psychiatrists, therapists, and counselors. Today we find it in wide circulation among

---

2. In fact, it was Dr. Jonathan Shay, MD, PhD—a pioneer and luminary in the effort to address the all too often catastrophic inner wounds suffered by military men and women in conflict—who first entered this term into public discourse. His definition of moral injury—"betrayal of 'what's right' in a high-stakes situation by someone who holds power"—was much more inclusive than that operative in most public forums today. What has been lost in this common bracketing of moral injury is a matter of foundational importance and of central concern to Dr. Shay: the corrosive abuse of power within the military, involving a culture of what he has labeled "leadership malpractice." While I share Dr. Shay's concern here, it is admittedly not the focus of this book and is a subject that I am in no way qualified to address. I can, however, urge the reader to explore his seminal discussion of moral injury in *Odysseus in America: Combat Trauma and the Trials of Homecoming.*

veterans and their professional caregivers, as well as in psychiatric journals, government reports, church pulpits, and the national media. More to our present purpose, it facilitates an inquiry and discussion such as this one, providing a common point of entry into a place that is both dark and painful, a place where many veterans find themselves suffering in confusion and despair, a place where nearly everyone else is reluctant to go. "Moral injury" has most commonly come to mean the transgression, the violation, of what is right, what one has long held to be sacred—a core belief or moral code—and thus wounding or, in the extreme, mortally wounding the psyche, soul, or one's humanity. As with so many concepts for which definitions fall short, moral injury is most clearly seen and understood in stories.

The story to which we first turn to illustrate and understand moral injury is but one of countless tragic stories of war and return, past and present. It is also a possibly familiar story made public in a number of media accounts and notably featured in a recent (2011) documentary titled *Wartorn 1861–2010*. It is the heartbreaking story of Noah Pierce[3] who, with his mother's reluctant consent, enlisted in the U.S. Army at the age of seventeen and less than two years later found himself in the vanguard of the March 2003 Iraq invasion. Four years later he sat alone in his pickup truck in Gilbert, Minnesota, put a gun to his head, and ended the life that had for him become unendurable. Scribbled on the back of an NRA pistol-safety certificate were these words to his mother:

> Mom, I am so sorry. My life has been hell since March 2003 when I was part of the Iraq invasion. . . . I am freeing myself from the desert once and for all. . . . I am not a good person. I have done bad things. I have taken lives. Now it's time to take mine.[4]

In the words of a close family friend, Noah was "too sensitive" and "too caring" to go to war and ever come back whole. Those words proved prophetic. He came back different, darkened, broken, haunted. In his letters home, Noah had described many of the "bad things" that he had witnessed and done in Iraq, as fear turned to anger and anger turned to hatred. He took some lives by accident, like the child he crushed under his Bradley Fighting Vehicle, but others he took deliberately, like the unarmed man he shot in the forehead at point-blank range or the last person he killed, a

---

3. Unless otherwise attributed, in the ensuing discussion of Noah Pierce, I am reliant upon Gilbertson, "The Life and Lonely Death of Noah Pierce."

4. See Alpert and Goosenberg, *Wartorn*.

doctor, at a checkpoint. "He couldn't forgive himself for some of the things he did," explains his mother:

> And he thought of himself as a murderer, and a bad person, because he still had the urge to hurt people, kill people. The United States Army turned my son into a killer. They trained him to kill to protect others. They forgot to un-train him, to take that urge to kill away from him.[5]

Noah Pierce was not a war criminal, only a warrior who served his country as well as he knew how. After two deployments in Iraq he was given an honorable discharge from the army and returned home to a grateful nation. In the eyes of those who knew little or nothing of what he knew, he was a hero, an accolade he wanted no part of. "So tell me," he wrote to his mother while still in Iraq, "how we are heroes."[6] Until he shot himself, Noah Pierce bore no physical wound, no sign of injury. His kind of wound, his mother explains, "kills you from the inside out."[7] His kind of wound is what we mean by moral injury, and although this book will not pretend to probe the psychological layers of moral injury, much less prescribe therapies for its healing, it will reveal its roots. And to do that we must trace the Western history of moral injury in war back to its recorded beginnings in ancient Greece and follow its path through the Christian centuries to modern Europe and contemporary America.

The tragedy of Noah Pierce finds an early precursor in a war drama written and enacted twenty-five centuries ago about a war that was already at the time ancient history. I have in mind a seldom read and still more seldom staged play entitled *Philoctetes* that the classical Greek playwright Sophocles wrote in his old age, at eighty-seven to be exact, after a long life not only in the theater of Dionysus but also in the theater of war. He had so far survived several wars on Greek soil and served in at least two of them, twice elected to the rank of *strategos* or "general." This is to say that in depicting war and its wounds Sophocles knew well what he was talking about. More specifically, he could not have been a stranger to moral injury; for he knew firsthand the intimate face-to-face savagery of ancient warfare, especially the protracted Greek-on-Greek civil warfare of the Peloponnesian War, notorious for its indiscriminate brutality and civilian carnage.

5. Ibid.

6. Ibid.

7. Ibid.

As Sophocles composed and staged *Philoctetes*, the Peloponnesian War was in its twenty-second year. Although he set the action of the play in the hoary past of the Trojan War, Sophocles wrote to the current war that Athenians knew all too well. It was conventional and convenient for tragic playwrights to don the masks of myth and legend when confronting their contemporaries with inconvenient truths. The past was, or seemed, safe, even entertaining, until like a mirror it reflected its audience. Stories worth telling are like that. They take us up and away into another reality before bringing us back to ourselves, eyes wide open. They promise escape, and give us truth instead. "The truth," wrote the Greek philosopher Heraclitus, "likes to hide."[8] And we surely like to hide from it. But there was no hiding from truth in the theater, the *theatron,* as the Greeks called it, which meant "the seeing place, the place of vision."

When the curtain, as it were, lifts on *Philoctetes,* the Trojan War is well into its tenth year, and for the Greeks it appears unwinnable. The dead may not yet outnumber the living, but they surely put them to shame. The best of the Greeks, their shining heroes, lie buried, while their lessers—most notably the politicians and posers—wander the Greek camp wondering what went wrong. This comes as no surprise to the wizened Philoctetes, who undoubtedly speaks for his maker when he says: "War never takes the bad man but by chance, the good man always" (436–37).[9] Nevertheless, at least according to the prophet Helenus, one chance remains for a Greek victory at Troy, and that chance is embodied in the bent and broken castaway, Philoctetes.

Greek victory at Troy, however, is far from our present concern and so is the full unfolding of *Philoctetes'* plotline. As it happens, the pivotal character of the play is not Philoctetes but rather a young boy named Neoptolemus, the son of the dead hero Achilles. He is the war's latest and most celebrated recruit, and by a twist of fate the war's outcome will depend on him. The fact is that he knows nothing about war, and he never really knew his illustrious father. He is as green as he is eager to go to war. His father's son, he wants to do his part. The tragedy is that his honorable, if irascible, father is no longer alive to teach him his part. Instead, the ever-scheming Odysseus steps in and pretends to fill a father's shoes. Odysseus sees only

8. Heraclitus, fragment 123, in Kirk and Raven, *Presocratic Philosophers,* 193. Translation mine.

9. These and subsequent numbers in parentheses indicate line numbers in the David Grene translation of Sophocles' *Philoctetes.*

opportunity in Neoptolemus' innocence and inexperience. He knows he can use him to accomplish his end, and the boy will be none the wiser until it is too late for him to know better.

The drama of Philoctetes is about betrayal and violation and the moral pain and confusion they leave in their wake. It is enough for us to know that the young Neoptolemus no sooner reports for duty than he is assigned a mission by Odysseus that contradicts his moral code, his sense of what is right, violates everything he has been taught about honor. A mere boy, fresh from the best of homes, he is well reared but as yet untested. This is his first test in an unfamiliar world where his deeds, not his words, will define him. His premonition and fear are that what he does now will determine his character, his direction in life. Odysseus, for his part, is no fool. He knows what the boy before him is feeling and fearing. Like Sophocles, Odysseus may even recognize himself in Neoptolemus, remembering a moment long ago when he had the same fears. A man of many words and few deeds, a man with a "shabby slit-eyed soul" (1013), Odysseus knows just what to say:

> I know, young man, it is not your natural bent
> To say such things nor to contrive such mischief.
> But the prize of victory is pleasant to win.
> Bear up: another time we shall prove honest.
> For one brief shameless portion of a day
> Give me yourself, and then for all the rest
> You may be called most scrupulous of men. (79–85)

In response, Neoptolemus proves no match for his mentor. He tries to hold his moral ground but soon yields, all but inevitably. "I recognize," he admits to Odysseus, "that I was sent with you to follow your instructions. I am loath to have you call me a traitor" (93–95). His moral principles are reduced to personal preferences, and Odysseus, whose confessed aim "in everything is to win" (1052), does just that here. He owns Neoptolemus for the moment, and the moment is all he needs.

Later in the play, when Neoptolemus comes to realize the wrong he has done and its consequences, he tries to retrace his steps and undo his own deed. What he discovers is that character once relinquished is not easily reclaimed. Life is no pawnshop. He is wounded, but the wound in this case is self-inflicted. The malaise he suffers is that of moral injury, which he self-diagnoses and describes in these timeless words: "All is disgust when one leaves his own nature and does things that misfit it" (902–3). We will return to these words in a moment, for they deserve close scrutiny and promise crucial insight. In the short space of the play, unfolding across a single day, we witness Neoptolemus the boy become Neoptolemus the veteran, who followed orders, did what needed to be done, bowed to what in the play is called a great, compelling necessity, and played his part in the Greek victory at Troy. At the same time, however, he leaves the audience and us with an unanswered and perhaps unanswerable question: "Is there no place, then, for repentance?" (1270).

We may question or at least wonder at the use of the word "repentance" here. Others take the Greek word in question to point to something more like "a change of mind." Either way, what Neoptolemus wants is to be able to start over, to reverse himself, to take back what he did and to do something else instead. "Repentance" suggests remorse and an accompanying effort to "make up" or to compensate for a wrong done. But the Greek word here—*metagnōnai*—is closer to "make over" than to "make up." Neoptolemus doesn't want to accept that what is done is done. Rather than move on, he wants to move back. Inexperienced to the point of naiveté, he hasn't yet fully accepted that time only flows in one direction. To realize fully what he is thinking and suffering we will need to go back now, as we said we would, and examine more closely his earlier lament: "All is disgust when one leaves his own nature and does things that misfit it."

The key word and concept here is "nature" (*phusis*). By "his own nature" Neoptolemus could presumably mean "human nature," his nature as a human being, or he could be referring to his own personal nature or character. In other words, when he did what he did and now regrets, Neoptolemus either forgot *what* he was or *who* he was or both. His action, in one or both senses, was "unnatural" to him and has brought with it a feeling of inner repulsion. This desperate complaint of inner repulsion and its root cause are nothing peculiar to Neoptolemus and his times. It is what we mean today by "moral injury," which is to say that Neoptolemus is not alone in his pain. But how is it that we can violate our own nature? "Human nature" has come to mean whatever we find human beings doing; and who today would claim that individuals have natures of their own? In order to understand Neoptolemus' pain (and our own) and not just feel it, we need to take a strategically brief excursion into Greek philosophy and, more specifically, into the "nature of nature" or the meaning of *phusis* as Sophocles likely understood it. This will be the first of many times we need to pause our central narrative in order to quarry a concept or idea that will prove essential to the historical and theological argument at the core of this book.

In the writings of Plato and Aristotle, the *phusis* or "nature" of any-thing referred to the full arc of its unfolding from seed to fruition, from birth to full being. It was a term that had to do with the "becoming" of anything across time, whether it be an art form like tragic drama, a tree like the oak, a disease like cholera, or an animal such as the elephant. Each has its own germinal beginning, its stages of development or growth, and its own proper fullness or end. Aristotle comments on how, in a world of becoming, a world like ours of motion and change, everything has its own *energeia*, its own inner being-at-work, its own direction and momentum. Fire, he says, rises when ignited, whereas stones, when released from the hand that holds them, fall. Acorns become oak trees, never elephants. All very obvious, all common sense, until we turn to human being. In the case of human being, he suggests, we need to picture an archer. He notches his arrow, draws his bow, aims, and releases the shaft to take its course. It's all in the drawing of the bow, and of course the aim. They will determine the arrow's arc, its direction and reach. The point here is that the archer pos-sesses a full and heady freedom to choose the arrow's path, just as human beings may and must choose their direction in life. What are the options to choose from? If we look around, we see them. They span, says Plato, the full expanse from heaven to hell, pointing out that some human beings are the gentlest, kindest creatures on the face of the earth, while others outdo the wildest animals in savagery and the most demented demons in their dark ways. The choice, he would say, is ours. Such is the burden and blessing of human freedom.

So is that it? Human nature is nothing but unfettered freedom of choice? Not according to Aristotle. We need to go back to the archer and notice that he has only one arrow, just as each of us has only one life. This is to say that our freedom is lost in the moment it is exercised. When the arrow leaves the bow it escapes the archer's control, which only a moment before was total. But surely in the case of our lives, it doesn't all happen so fast, in an instant. No, but it happens sooner than we would like. It hap-pens in youth, according to Aristotle, as soon as we begin to act and make choices. He describes the process as a circle, in which action shapes char-acter and character shapes action. In others words, we shape who we are by our actions and after a while we act more and more in accord with who we are. When we tell lies we become liars, and liars soon find that lies come more easily to them than the truth. The opposite is the case for those who commit themselves to telling the truth. After a while, after many turns of this wheel, habits are formed and our "character" takes full shape. Here again, in the word we have a telling image of the reality at hand. The Greek word *charakter* refers to an impression stamped into a coin or a seal cut or pressed into wood or wax. It is "fixed" once and for all, not readily altered or removed without injury or damage. Later in the history of thought, in late antiquity and the Middle Ages, this reality is referred to as "second nature," which is not to be confused with first nature or human nature.

So what is "human nature" and where does it come in? According to Plato and Aristotle it is always there, from the beginning, as it were, an idea that could easily stop us in our tracks. Fortunately, all that we need to keep in mind at this point in our discussion is that human nature, as it was once and wisely understood, is not like the nature of anything else. It doesn't account for the way people act or for the lives they live. Remember the archer and his freedom. Human nature doesn't determine *what* we do, it only determines what we *ought* to do. It describes our moral limits or boundaries, which we are free to cross but not without consequences. It means our freedom is not without its limits. As soon as we begin to become aware of ourselves, our world, and our possibilities, we discover that we are able to do more and other than we ought to do. The appeal here to "limits" is not to any civic or social law, laid down by states or sovereigns, but rather to a law that we only come to know from within and then perhaps only when we transgress it, as Neoptolemus did. We experience it as disgust, contempt, and despair at having violated something at our core, either our human core or our personal core or quite probably both. "Native and indwelling in every soul is a cross-examiner . . . which is our accuser and our judge,"[10] asserts Philo, and we know this accuser by different names. Perhaps most often we see him or her in the mirror.

Make no mistake, the portrait of Neoptolemus that Sophocles preserved in *Philoctetes* is not the whole story of the infamous son of Achilles. It is a snapshot of a moment, suspended in time, when a kind and compassionate boy from the best of homes, answering his "nation's" call and honoring the memory of his fallen father, came of age, went off to war, followed orders, did the necessary, lost his soul, and tried in vain to get it back. Others tell the rest of the story—how Neoptolemus (also known as "Pyrrhus") played a decisive role in the Greek victory at Troy and at the same

10. Philo Judaeus, *Decalogue*, 87, cited in Konstan, *Before Forgiveness*.

time disfigured his own and his family's legacy with sacrilege and atrocity. It was he who slew the aged Priam as he clung to the family altar, leaving his remains where they lay as food scraps for the household hounds. It was he too who tore the child Astyanax, son of Hector, from his mother's arms and hurled him from the city's walls. Later, he slit the throat of Astyanax's sister, Polyxena, over his own father's burial mound, supposedly because Achilles' ghost had cried out in thirst for her blood. After all of that we hear no more of his inner doubts or disgust. Instead, there are conflicting versions of his post-war feats and his eventual violent death, but not before he slept with, among others, Hector's widow and Helen's daughter, his seed in time making its way down to help fashion another boy-become-conqueror, named Alexander, who also never knew when to stop.

Neoptolemus is not just a famous face from the past. His story is not only a *Greek* tragedy. Even his name, *neo-p(t)olemus,* "new war," suggests that he may not be easy to consign to antiquity. Admittedly, he's an extreme case. The Greeks were fond of extremes, no matter how fervently they preached moderation.

When young veterans, like Neoptolemus or Noah Pierce, experience their first taste of war and its demands, what is it that they so often experience as having violated their nature, stolen their humanity, killed their souls, and made them criminals? What has been their crime? The simplest answer to this may have been given long ago by Amphitryon to his young son Herakles, fresh from battle, crazed and bent on death:

> O child what is happening to you?
> Where have you left us and gone to?
> You're raving and possessed. Why? It must be the killing
> you've just done. You still have their blood on you . . . in you.[11]

There is no doubt regarding the criminality of killing in everyday life. The criminality of killing in war, on the other hand, is usually considered less problematic. War issues waivers to its participants, free passes, as it were, to take each other's lives with impunity; but it has never been that simple, as we shall see when we consider the history of this problem, the problem of legal or justified, much less celebrated, killing. Our Western Theories and Rules of Just War and Moral Murder, the ones we still invoke to silence our deepest misgivings over shedding blood, have from the

---

11. Euripides, *Herakles,* lines 963–64. For a full translation and discussion of Euripides' *Herakles,* see Meagher, *Herakles Gone Mad.*

outset stood on soft soil. As we shall soon see, in the early centuries of the Common Era they emerged amidst fierce debate, and long after that, well into the medieval period, they had their earnest if ineffectual doubters and defectors. Oddly, that debate seems moot in our day. Granted, the legitimacy of this or that particular war may still be challenged, but the fact that war admits of legitimacy goes without saying. More than any other event in modern memory, World War II represents the capstone (or perhaps the gravestone) of the Just War Tradition. It makes the needed case and silences all but the most radical dissent. It proves, for nearly everyone, at least in Europe and the United States, that there is such a thing as a just war, a good war, a war that can be waged without scruples. In his highly touted book *The Unforgiving Minute: A Soldier's Education,*[12] West Point graduate and Rhodes Scholar Craig Mullaney relates how during his basic training, when he struggled to reconcile his moral code and religious upbringing with the fact that he was being trained to kill and to order others to do the same, he sought out his Catholic chaplain, who put his qualms to rest by asking, "Do you believe in a just war?" "I think so, Father," responded Mullaney, adding, "Like World War II?" "Believe" is the operative word here. One faith, it seems, may be used to trump another. The proof for the existence not of God but of just war is clearly the "Good War," the war against Hitler and Hirohito, the war against evil; and the accompanying assumption that needs no proof is that a war against evil cannot possibly be itself evil.

We are already ahead of ourselves at this point in our examination of just war, but it is important from the start to take note of one or two realities that are surprisingly often overlooked in the rush to war and in the rush, afterwards, to forget it. For one, we need to realize that war, as envisioned in just war theory—originally and for nearly two millennia—bore little or no resemblance to the wars that we have known in the last century. Before there was the "Good War" there was the "Great War," which ushered in what has rightfully been called the age of massacre. The scale and savagery of warfare as witnessed in the trenches of northern Europe from 1914 to 1918 shocked the world—420,000 British dead and another 60,000 killed on the first day of the Battle of the Somme. By the end of the war, the British had lost a generation, nearly 800,000 men, the majority of them upper-class, privileged, and finely educated. Meanwhile, the French lost a million men and the Germans closer to two million. The American dead numbered far fewer, just over 120,000, more than half of these from disease rather

12. Mullaney, *Unforgiving Minute,* 30–32.

than combat. Words did not and do not come easily to describe or comprehend such slaughter. All the same, as the savage harvest of World War I was underway, Sigmund Freud offered this less than prescient comment in his *Reflections on War and Death*:

> When the fierce struggle of this war will have reached a decision every victorious warrior will joyfully and without delay return home to his wife and children, undisturbed by thoughts of the enemy he has killed either at close quarters or with weapons operating at a distance.[13]

What would assure so untroubled a homecoming for veterans of the Great War, as Freud saw it, was the happy fact that they, like all "civilized" men, had lost their "ethical delicacy of feeling." Savage men, he explained, lived in fear of the men they murdered—of their lingering vengeful spirits, that is—whereas modern men knew better than to allow the past to haunt them. To their credit and to their agony, however, Freud underestimated the consciences of the men and women who returned from the trenches and the killing fields of the Great War and of every war since. What they saw and suffered and especially what they did in war came home with them and darkened the remainder of their days.

A generation later, following the horror of the Great War, the Good War proved immeasurably more horrific. The ranks of its countless dead dwarfed those of World War I. The age of massacre had gained momentum. What was new, however, was the indiscriminate massacre of civilians. Only a small fraction of the dead in the Good War, the deadliest conflict in history, had borne arms. They were mere kindling and fuel for the fire that fell on them, mostly from the sky. The traditional ratio of civilian to combatant deaths in war was turned on end, apparently for the indefinite future. President Obama acknowledged but understated this fact when, again in his Nobel speech, he pointed out that "in today's wars, many more civilians are killed than soldiers."[14] Setting aside questions of justice, it is questionable whether the wars of the last century as well as our own more recent conflicts can, without reservation, be called "war" at all. By definition, writes the eminent theorist and historian of war Martin Van Creveld,

> war does not consist simply of a situation where one person or group puts the other to death . . . ; rather, it begins at that point

13. Freud, *Reflections on War and Death*, 20–21.
14. Obama, "Nobel."

where inflicting mortal injury becomes reciprocal, an activity known as fighting. . . . In any war, the readiness to suffer and die, as well as to kill, represents the single most important factor.[15]

Killing without personal risk is something else and requires another name, assassination or execution, but that thought takes us where we are not yet prepared to go in this discussion. All we can say for now is that it is no wonder that those who witness such killing firsthand, whether they engage in it or not, are haunted to the end of their days by the memories of what they have seen.

In recent years we in the United States have found ourselves once again mired in war, two wars in fact, of longer duration than either of the world wars of the twentieth century. While it is all too easy for civilians to lose track of the passage of time, the loss of life, and the devastation of spirit and soul in our current conflicts, those who fight them for us cannot but keep a precise, inner tally of their cost. As we have already seen, the most invisible and silent cost is the one dismissed by Freud—the violated conscience—invisible because hidden, silent because silenced. Breaking that silence we again hear—this time from our veterans—the timeless voice of Neoptolemus, asking, "Is there no place, then, for repentance?"

In an age, like ours, of civilian massacre, knee-deep in blood, it is neither premature nor unreasonable to wonder if we have lost our way, as a nation and as a world. Do we any longer know what we are doing in sending our young men and women into all but unthinkable situations to do what we would never do and would rather not know about, except as it is eventually packaged for general consumption, as news or entertainment? This much we do know—that wars are not over when they're over. They leave behind wreckage and wounds. Warriors bring their war home with them, not like a tan acquired on holiday but like a secret they wish they hadn't been told.

What about that secret? After the wars of the twentieth century—especially those wars labeled "great" and "good"—the common wisdom passed on to veterans from every side regarding what they knew and others could not know was clichéd: "let it go," "leave it alone and it will leave you alone," "leave it behind and it will stay there; just move on." All this made—and makes—perfect sense, except to veterans. "Alone" . . . "behind" . . . how convenient! To the uninitiated: common sense. To the warrior come home: silent betrayal.

15. Van Creveld, *Transformation*, 160.

Why betrayal? What's wrong with forgetting what we wish we had never learned? Why not "sweet oblivion"? Re-enter the ancients, because they have something to say that perhaps we have not heard yet or thought about lately.

Curiously, the word for "the past" in ancient Greek means that which we face, and the word for "the future" means that which is behind our back. What sense, we ask, does that make? Don't we walk into the future with our back to the past? In that case, however, as the Greeks see it, we are walking blind. Yes, of course, our eyes face forward—time's inevitable direction and ours as well. But, as we do so, as we move through the time of our lives, it's the past that we can see and the future to which we are blind. As Homer describes it, the future and, inevitably, death stalk us from behind, our blind side. We cannot see death coming, but we know it is. The fact is that when we leave our past behind—forgetting it or banishing it—like Oedipus, we pluck out our own eyes and start over, not knowing who we are or what we are doing. Such oblivion is never truly sweet, only foolish. What I propose, then, in this book is to shed light on the present and to provide some guidance for the future by walking into the past. The walk I propose, however, is no idle ramble, but rather a strategic tracing of the roots and branches of our Western understanding of war and, more pointedly, of just war and moral injury. The past, after all, is what we can know and is at the same time what we cannot afford not to know.

2

Ancient Greece

Warriors and Lovers

T HE GREEKS, OR MORE specifically Homer, gave us in the West our earliest literary taste of war and with it our first words and concepts for understanding and dealing with war's contradictions. It is all but a truism among military historians that the ancient Greeks invented and defined the "Western way of war." That may be, but an even more immediate link to the present might be found in the concept and practice of "battlemind," a current buzzword in the U.S. Army meant to convey the inner core of the ideal warrior, what Homer might call his *thumos*, an embodied life-and-death force all but defined by such figures as Achilles and Hector, two of the human planets fated to collide in the *Iliad*, arguably the greatest war story ever written. While the historical accuracy of Homer's masterwork has been and will be debated until the world runs out of words, its "truth," I would argue, has never been seriously in question. "A true war story, if truly told," writes Vietnam combat veteran Tim O'Brien, "makes the stomach believe."[1] And the *Iliad* has been doing that, for modern as well as for ancient warriors, from the day it was first sung. General George Patton drank in Homer as a boy, and Alexander the Great—hardly more than a boy when he set out to conquer the world—slept with his copy of the *Iliad* under his pillow. More recently, U.S. senators and noted war

---

1. O'Brien, *Things They Carried*, 78.

veterans Max Cleland and John McCain, in their foreword to Jonathan Shay's contemporary classic, *Odysseus in America*, write,

> Those of us who have witnessed, taken part in, and suffered the tragedies of war know that the ancient Greek epics offer compelling insights into our own experiences. In the *Iliad*, an epic of war, and the *Odyssey*, an epic of a veteran's attempt to get home, Homer speaks as one who has "been there."[2]

The *Iliad* has been, across the centuries, then, for warriors and veterans, one of "the things they carried," one of the stories they lived, killed, and died with, one of the stories that made sense to them, one of the stories that made sense *of* them. Again we turn to the words of Tim O'Brien, author of *The Things They Carried*:

> That's what stories are for. Stories are for joining the past to the future. Stories are for those late hours in the night when you can't remember how you got from where you were to where you are. Stories are for eternity, when memory is erased, when there is nothing to remember except the story.[3]

The *Iliad* is indeed a bridge that helps us understand how we got where we are today, as warriors and as a nation at war. We see in it the germ, the seed, the *phusis*, to recall an earlier discussion, of what we know and experience today. We may well study it for much the same reason that midshipmen at the U.S. Naval Academy learn sailing—to touch not the old but the timeless, before it is gone.

For this reason and more we begin on the battlefield of Troy as the *Iliad* allows us to envision it. We see two "cities" at war, the one built of stone and brick and the other of wood. The city of stone with its legendary battlements and gates is, of course, towering Troy, while the "city" of wood is merely the makeshift camp of the invading Greek armada, comprised of a thousand beached ships and countless jerry-rigged shelters, girded by defensive earthworks and wooden palisades. Between these two cities stretches the Trojan plain, the killing fields, where the two armies—Trojan and Greek—meet in battle. Victory for the Greeks would mean their breaching the walls of Troy and setting the city ablaze, whereas a Trojan victory would mean their overrunning the Greek encampment and burning the ships. In the one case, the Trojans lose their homes, and in the other

2. Shay, *Odysseus in America*, xi.
3. O'Brien, *Things They Carried*, 38.

the Greeks lose their homecomings. In either case, innumerable Greek and Trojans lose their lives.

From the start, then, at very first glance, we grasp that the stakes are high for both sides. The Greek warriors have come to kill and to risk being killed in order to breach the walls of Troy, and the Trojans know only too well the consequences of defeat for them and for their families; so they will spare no lives—neither the Greeks' nor their own—to assure that that does not happen. This fight, in other words, is a war in the strictest sense—balanced and reciprocal. It is a contest so balanced, in fact, that it rages on through its tenth year without a clear winner. This is the back-and-forth way of war, as the war god Ares' epithet or nickname describes: *alloprosallos*, "leaning first this way, then that way." As in sports, so also in war, "momentum" is a fickle force. The balanced nature of the Trojan War, as Homer gives it to us, goes even further. The two sides are also morally balanced. Neither side is favored, much less demonized. Each small conquest is both celebrated and suffered, each loss of life is acknowledged, "conqueror and conquered are brothers in the same distress."[4] "No man is set above or below the condition common to all men," comments Simone Weil, "whatever is destroyed is regretted."[5] The poem ends with two funerals—one for Patroklos, the most beloved of the Greeks, and the other for Hector, the most beloved of the Trojans—and we weep equally for both. What we witness in this ancient war story, so rare that we can't miss it, is the moral equality of the enemies. "There may be, unknown to us," writes Simone Weil, "other expressions of the extraordinary sense of equity which breathes through the *Iliad*; certainly it has not been imitated. One is barely aware that the poet is a Greek and not a Trojan . . . this poem is a miracle."[6]

Another fact of this war that we cannot fail to notice is the remarkable rarity of personal hatred on or off the battlefield of Troy. Apparently, the willingness to kill in war need not rest on personal loathing or contempt for, much less dehumanization of, the other. In war, the Greeks made a linguistic and conceptual distinction between a *polemios* and an *ekhthros*. The former is a military foe, an opponent on the field of battle. He is the person I am there to kill, or to be killed by, as the case may be. We might have been neighbors last month and we might again be neighbors next month, but today we find ourselves on opposite sides of a line that we personally have

4. Weil, *Iliad*, 19.

5. Ibid., 30.

6. Ibid., 32–33.

not drawn. Not so with the *ekhthros*, my personal enemy, for whom I have a deep contempt and hatred, a malice that is most often fully mutual. We find this too in the *Iliad*, between Menelaus and Paris, Achilles and Agamemnon, and, to be sure, Achilles and Hector. In these last two, the enmity and hatred run so deep and extend so far that they are disfigured by it. To these two alone, of all the warriors at Troy, Homer attributes *lyssa* or "battle madness." In a dog or wolf, the same term is used to indicate rabies. In a word, Achilles and Hector are rabid in their rage. They are the war's only two designated and diagnosed berserkers; and of the two, it is Achilles who, for a time, leaves his humanity far behind, so far behind that he hungers for Hector's raw flesh, though in the end he can't bring himself to sit down to the meal he has made. Even the inhuman rage of Achilles finally passes, and he finds himself able to respect the same corpse that he once defiled and hand it over to Hector's father Priam, with an embrace and with tears.

Returning to the Greeks and Trojans in conflict, we ask what if not hatred has set these two cities or peoples at such deadly odds, to wage a war seemingly without end? What or who, in short, is the *causa belli*, the provocation or prize that has ignited and sustained this conflict? Her name, everyone knows, is Helen. This is a war over a woman. Before there was consuming hate or enmity, there was overwhelming desire, sexual desire or longing (*pothos*), for the most beautiful woman in the world, the polestar of all male longing. This is what we are told and expected to take in, not only in this war poem but also in the *Odyssey*, where the great concluding battle or massacre of the epic is fought over Penelope, a very different sort of woman and wife from Helen, but apparently every bit as compelling and provocative of lethal rivalry. The truth is, however, that not only in the Greek tradition are the greatest of wars fought over the most beautiful of women. Even a glance at the two monumental epics of ancient India—the *Mahabharata* and the *Ramayana*—reveals that each culminates in a great war fought over a woman of surpassing, luminous, irresistible beauty, a queen abducted and requiring to be retrieved at any cost. The intriguing parallels between these two vast Sanskrit epics and the Homeric poems, so far from ending, only begin with the all but divine women at their core; but, if we are to get on with our discussion of the *Iliad*, this must remain a road untaken.[7]

7. There are many such relevant and intriguing side roads to be explored. For example, the closest ancient East Mediterranean cousin to the *Iliad* may be the Ugaritic *Epic of Kirta* in which another great war is waged over a woman, this time Hurriya, daughter of the king of Udm, who is abducted by Kirta, a hero-king of ancient Canaan. This early

Killing from the Inside Out

The story of how Helen came to be the cause of the Trojan War is well known. Whether she ran off from her husband willingly or went under force, Menelaus, her wronged mate, holds Paris, Prince of Troy, responsible. Even so, the war over Helen is not the only game going in the *Iliad*. There are, in fact, two major conflicts in the poem. In addition to the "hot war" waged between the Greeks and Trojans, there is a "cold war" waged between Achilles and Agamemnon, and this war too is over a beautiful woman, the "spear-prize" Briseis, stolen from Achilles by Agamemnon, to compensate for the seizure of still another stunner, golden Chryseis. This latter war would not have been "cold" or bloodless, had it not been for the timely intervention of Athena, who stayed the sword-arm of Achilles when he would have otherwise put a rapid end to the arrogant and overreaching warlord Agamemnon.

What can we say about the others, the innumerable and mostly unnamed Greeks willing to kill and die in what appears to be no more than a blood feud between two men claiming title to the same woman? Is vicarious jealousy and sex enough to marshal and motivate tens of thousands of other Greeks, whose wives lie at home in empty beds, to go to war and stay there for ten years? These hapless grunts will likely never set eyes on Helen much less linger with her in love. Like most other recruits and conscripts in the ancient world and later, they are there for the loot. Ancient wars were seldom fought over real estate. The spoils of war were what you as a victor could carry away with you—portable treasure, the plunder of battle divvied up and doled out according to rank, prowess, and the whims of the warlord. We witness in the *Iliad* that these war prizes included such items as gold, horses, cauldrons and cooking tripods, bronze-tipped spears and armor, finely crafted swords, crested helmets, and—best of all spear-prizes—women. We are somehow expected to believe that these are what the ordinary invader at Troy killed and died for. Clearly, however, the fine horses, glittering gold, and most desirable women would never go to the common nameless human fodder who would perish at Troy, or not, either way without notice. No wonder morale became an issue and reached a crisis point when, given a chance, the Greek troops ran for their ships. It was the aged but still astute Nestor who found the right chiding words to turn them around and set them back on task by calling out,

---

poem might even have served as a partial model for the *Iliad*.

> No man here should be in a hurry to go home
> Until he has spent the night with some Trojan's wife
> As revenge for Helen's struggles and groans.[8]

Put simply, there's a Helen behind those walls for every one of you. She may not be the match of Helen, but she's yours for the taking.

In war, then and all too often now, rape was assumed to be the lot of the losers and the first loot of the winners. A simple reminder of this was enough to stanch the en-masse desertion of the Greek army. Now every Greek at Troy was at war over a Helen of some size and shape, a woman to subdue and make his own, to take as "wife." Tellingly, the Greek word for wife—*damar*—comes from the verb *damao* or *damadzo,* which means to yoke, tame, conquer, rape, or kill. It is a violent word, describing a violent task. Women were seen as wild and "other"; they needed to be broken like horses rather than simply picked like flowers or harvested like grain. Wives, like slaves, though tamed, had to be watched. Once wild, always wild. Foreign cities too, like strange women, had to be taken by force. Illustrative of this is the fact that the same word—*kredemna*—stood for the walls of a city and the veils of its women. The breaching of a city's walls, then, was a symbolic act of rape, as was the stripping away of its women's veils. The one is a prelude to the other; for when a city (seen as feminine) is violated, the violation of its girls and women is only moments away.

We have again come face to face with the sexuality of war and conquest, whose many dimensions we have only begun to explore here. While our focus here is on Homer and the *Iliad,* it is important to note that the fusion of war and sex, the erotic character of violent conflict and conquest, is not confined to Bronze Age epics. To illustrate this, I will give a couple of examples from elsewhere in Greek history and literature. The first is from the Athenian historian Thucydides, himself a general, as he attempts to describe the admittedly deranged fervor of his city for the about-to-be-launched invasion of Sicily in the summer of 415 BCE, a fatal caper from which imperial Athens never fully recovered. Perhaps at something of a loss to describe the condition of the people of Athens at this point he tells how: "There was a passion for the enterprise which affected everyone alike."[9] The Greek text is a bit more graphic. It says that *eros* seized everyone, and that the object of this *eros* or erotic passion was the sailing, the expedition to

8. Homer, *Iliad,* 2.383–85.

9. Thucydides, *Peloponnesian War,* 6.24.3.

Troy. Put more bluntly, the city was "in heat" for the invasion, the latest expression of Athens' insatiable lust for empire.

The invasion of Sicily, we must understand, was sheer madness. Athens was in the seventeenth year of a protracted war, already waged on several fronts. The people's plate was full and they should have been by any measure war-weary to their bones. Instead, they were enflamed with desire (*eros*). Eros, in the Greek imagination, is more than a hormone, he is a god, at once a primordial deity, part of the essential architecture of existence, and at the same time the son of the sex goddess Aphrodite. His twin brother, Himeros, is the god of sexual desire, and as if this were not enough fire in one family's blood, these two have a third brother, Pothos, the god of sexual longing. To be sure, in art and legend, Eros enjoys a sometimes cute and endearing persona as Cupid, but more often than not he is a predatory force to be feared and best avoided. The chorus of young girls in Euripides' *Iphigenia at Aulis* know well that Eros is best taken in small doses:

> Blessed are those who sip the pleasures of Aphrodite
> Slowly, from a shallow cup.
> In her bed, peace of mind is a rare prize.
> Blessed is anyone who finds calm there,
> Where most are driven mad.
> Eros, the golden-haired boy with the bow,
> Has but two arrows in his quiver.
> The one brings bliss.
> The other casts a net of confusion
> And chaotic pain.
> Keep that boy and his arrows,
> I beg you, radiant lady,
> Far from me and from my bed.
> I pray for the middle path,
> For a tame love that knows its place.
> I want my share of Aphrodite.
> But no more.[10]

It is disconcerting how often Death (Thanatos) and Eros connive. Like Death, Eros stalks and takes down his prey, cutting their legs from under them. "With his venom irresistible and bittersweet," writes the poet Sappho,

10. Cited in Meagher, *Essential Euripides*, 339–40.

"that loosener of limbs, Love [Eros] reptile-like strikes me down."[11] Make no mistake, Eros and his brothers are often deadly. It's not only that those they afflict can die of lovesickness. There is also the fact that Eros drives people mad, separates them from all sense and reason, rendering them reckless and self-destructive. Witness the citizens of Athens on the eve of the Sicilian Expedition, aching in their beds, obsessed with images of a new conquest.

The playwright Aristophanes, another Athenian contemporary of Thucydides, had a similar take on the Sicilian expedition, attributing it to an insatiable erotic hunger for control, conquest, and empire. Shortly after the launching of the first of two armadas to Sicily, Aristophanes wrote and produced his comic masterpiece *The Birds*, in which two Athenians fantasize and then bring to fruition the grandest empire ever imagined, much less achieved, one that extends to the edges of their universe. In today's military super-speak, they have in their grasp "full-spectrum dominance." What is more to the point in our discussion here, Aristophanes casts the entire enterprise in sexual terms, as an erotic universal quest, or rather universal conquest, culminating in coitus, and no ordinary coitus at that. The play ends with a marriage amid the stars between an eros-driven Athenian and *Basileia* or "Empire," the "Bride of Heaven," whom the eminent classicist William Arrowsmith, in his translation of *The Birds*, calls "Miss Universe," a celestial Helen in the sky with diamonds.

The Athenians' partners and avian alter-egos in this play and its imperial scheme are the birds, the first of the gods, the primordial regents of the universe. They are the first-born sons of Love, hatched from the union of Eros and Chaos and often symbolically depicted as winged phalluses. They are never still, always reaching, always striving, gaping after the latest object of their ambition and desire. In this they are all too recognizably human. It was this realization that led the seventeenth-century philosopher Thomas Hobbes to assert that "in the first place I put for a generall inclination of all mankind, a perpetuall and restlesse desire of Power after power, that ceaseth onely in Death."[12] We are back to the familiarity, even the collusion, of eros with death, to the point that "it was a formal principle of Greek myth and literature that love and death [Eros and Thanatos] were two aspects of

---

11. Sappho, *Sappho*, 53.

12. Hobbes, *Leviathan*, I.11. Hobbes was no stranger to ancient Greek ideas. In fact, he produced the first English translation of Thucydides.

the same power."[13] And where do we find that power most blatantly and brutally wielded? On the battlefield, where winged Thanatos, in full panoply, makes his way through the carnage, gently lifting the dead into his arms and taking them away.

If Death, particularly violent death, has a face, it is War, and it should follow that Love would be the sworn enemy of both. At first glance War and Love would appear to be pure opposites, repulsive to each other. But we have seen for ourselves that that is not how the Greeks understood them. Instead, in Greek art, myth, and literature, we find them entangled, one minute incompatible and the next minute inseparable. We should not be all that surprised, then, to learn that they were on-again-off-again lovers. Ares the man-slaughterer, the god of war, the most hated of the Olympians, was drawn on more than one occasion to the most beautiful and beguiling goddess of all, Aphrodite, the embodiment of love. If not a match made in heaven, it still lit their mutual fire. But what of mere mortals, not only then but now? Before we go further, we may reasonably ask whether any of this resonates with warriors well beyond the shadow of antiquity. To this question, World War II veteran J. Glenn Gray writes,

> It is not without significance that the language of physical love and the language of battle have a large correspondence, and the phrase "the war of the sexes" can be rich in connotation. . . . The conquest of the sexual partner thus becomes very like the conquest of the enemy. . . . Observation of others and being honest about our own sensations must convince us that sexual passion in isolation and the lust for battle are closely akin. Such sexual passion and war have been married from the beginning.[14]

In describing the sexual act, the ancient physician Galen explains that "a very great pleasure is coupled with the exercise of the generative parts, and a raging desire precedes their use."[15] Regarding the climax that follows, the early Christian apologist Tertullian asks, "in that last breaking wave of delight, do we not feel something of our very soul go out from us?"[16] Love-making, in its climactic moments, is undeniably a convulsive act, but so too is killing, if it is up close and intimate. Both are orgasmic. André Malraux, in *Man's Fate*, gives us a vivid account of a young man's first kill.

13. Vermeule, *Aspects of Death*, 159.
14. Gray, *Warriors*, 66–68
15. Galen, *de usu partium* 14.9, cited in Brown, *Body and Society*, 17.
16. Tertullian, *de anima* 27.5, cited in Brown, *Body and Society*, 17.

Ch'en, a revolutionary soldier, steals into the silent bedroom of his sleeping victim and stands transfixed over him, knife in hand. Then, "with a blow that would have split a plank," he slashes through the mosquito netting and into the man below:

> Sensitive to the very tip of the blade, he felt the body rebound towards him, flung up by the springs of the bed. . . . A current of unbearable anguish passed between the corpse and himself, through the dagger, his stiffened arm, his aching shoulder, to the very depth of his chest, to his convulsive heart—the only thing moving in the room.[17]

Moments later, as he leaves the killing room and walks out into the world, he realizes (and remarks to himself), "What I have just done obviously doesn't show."[18] Like someone who has just had sex for the first time, he feels himself transformed. He will never be the same. Except to everyone else.

In civilian society, apart perhaps from wedding bands, there are no badges or insignia worn by those who have experienced sex. Determining who is a virgin and who is not is guesswork. Not so with combat in the army. Since 1941, the CIB or Combat Infantryman Badge clearly marks off those soldiers who have personally fought in active ground combat. Not to have earned this badge is, for a soldier, something akin to still being a virgin. As mentioned earlier, during and after the Vietnam War, U.S. combat veterans were often given to meet the war-related comments or questions of those who had not seen what they saw and done what they did with this dismissal: "If you didn't go, you don't know." There is no denying the truth in these words. And the same might be said to those who would prattle on about sex without ever having done it. In each case, there is a line, and there is only one way to cross it. I doubt that anyone ever forgets when or where he or she did just that.

Both warmaking and lovemaking are for the young, whose bodies are fit and whose passions run fast and furious. Aristotle, in comparing the character of the young man with that of mature or elderly men, points out that

> Young men have strong passions, and tend to gratify them indiscriminately. Of the bodily desires, it is the sexual by which they are most swayed and in which they show absence of self-control. . . . They are hot-tempered and quick-tempered, and apt

17. Malraux, *Man's Fate*, 11–12.

18. Ibid., 17.

to give way to their anger. . . . While they love honour they love victory still more. . . . Their hot tempers and hopeful dispositions make them more courageous than older men are; the hot temper prevents fear, and the hopeful disposition creates confidence; we cannot feel fear so long as we are feeling angry. . . . They would always rather do noble deeds than useful ones. . . . All their mistakes are in the direction of doing things excessively and vehemently. . . . They love too much and hate too much, and the same with everything else.[19]

It is no wonder that it is the young who fight our wars and who leap into bed to produce the next generation, made all the more crucial by the slaughter of war. "The Greeks were wise men," wrote Private Gray, from southern France in 1944, "when they mated the God of war with the goddess Aphrodite. The soldier must not only kill, he must give birth to new warriors."[20] The young warrior and lover knows all too well the alluring and addictive intensity of the bed and the battlefield, and how there is a happiness to be found in each. Virgins going to bed for the first time with a lover and warriors going into battle for the first time with the enemy know a similar excitement and anticipation. Both are tangible in this entry from the war diary of Ernst Juenger:

The great moment had come. The curtain of fire lifted from the front trenches. We stood up.

With a mixture of feelings, evoked by bloodthirstiness, rage, and intoxication, we moved in step, ponderously but irresistibly toward the enemy lines. I was well ahead of the company, followed by Vinke and a one-year veteran named Haake. My right hand embraced the shaft of my pistol, my left a riding stick of bamboo cane. I was boiling with a mad rage, which had taken hold of me and all the others in an incomprehensible fashion. The overwhelming wish to kill gave wings to my feet. Rage pressed bitter tears from my eyes.

The monstrous desire for annihilation, which hovered over the battlefield, thickened the brains of the men and submerged them in red fog. We called to each other in sobs and stammered disconnected sentences. A neutral observer might have perhaps believed that we were seized by an excess of happiness.[21]

19. Aristotle, *Rhetoric* II.12.
20. Gray, *Warriors*, 59.
21. Quoted in ibid., 52.

Karl Marlantes, drawing on his own experience half a century later as a Marine in the central highlands of Vietnam, confirms the same intoxicated rage and thrill of battle and explains that "in combat you are already over some edge. You are in a fierce state where there is a primitive and savage joy in doing in your enemy."[22]

Now, with the assurance that the past is never simply past and that a dialogue with the past is truly possible and fruitful, we return to the battlefield of Troy for a closer look at the character of combat revealed there, or, more precisely, in the lines of Homer's poem. We have already noted that in the *Iliad* each army has its base or "city" from which it sallies forth to do battle in the open plain. Once there, we notice further that there are, as in any war, front lines and rear guards. Some warriors are far closer to the fighting than others—some in the thick of it, some hanging back in relative safety. There are those too, in fact, who may only rarely if ever leave the security of Troy's walls or the Greeks' coastal bulwarks. In this category, apart from women, children, and the aged, there are the cooks, the healers, the priests, and others whose role is not to bear arms. Then there are the archers, who are combatants, killers in fact, but whose war-craft is somehow suspect, even disdainful. We can hear the disdain in which archers were held in these words of Diomedes, hurled back at Paris who had just wounded him with an arrow shot from safe concealment:

> You sissy, curly-haired pimp of a bowman!
> Why don't you come down and fight me man to man
> And see how far your bow and arrow get you?
> Boasting because you scratched my foot!
> I might as well have been hit by a woman
> Or an imbecile child.[23]

It is not that they are not deadly, because they are in fact quite deadly. Each side turns to their archers[24] to take out, for instance, an otherwise all but invincible foe. Godlike Achilles, after all, eventually falls to an archer's shaft, as does Paris. Archers kill, but they kill remotely, from a safe distance. There is little mutuality of risk in their warmaking. They often kill, but they are only rarely killed. Admittedly, the range and anonymity of a Bronze Age

22. Marlantes, *What It Is Like*, 30.

23. Homer, *Iliad*, 11.408–13.

24. In the *Iliad*, we learn of only two regular archers by name—Greek Teucer and Trojan Paris. Neither dies in the course of the poem.

arrow were not those of today's artillery shells, "smart" bombs, or cruise missiles, to say nothing of predator drones whose pilots sit thousands of miles from the point of actual attack. Then and now, "killing in war isn't always the morally clean 'it was them or me' situation which we so often hear about. . . . The more technically sophisticated we get, in fact, the less common this situation will become, and the more problematic the morality."[25] The bows employed at Troy were not, by our standards, sophisticated weapons, but they were sophisticated enough for ancient Greeks to be uneasy about using them to kill each other, when it involved little or no personal risk for the killer. Put simply, the Greeks had a determined disdain for remote forms of warfare. Like the samurai of Japan, Greek warriors found the measure of themselves and of others in close combat, eye to eye, hand to hand. They died in each others' arms. Killing remotely, without risk, was not what war was about; it was, instead, *phonos*—slaughter or murder—and there was no honor to be found nor glory to be won in that. There was a ritual of battle to be observed in war, and it is to that ritual we now turn.

Nearly all of the several hundred warriors whose deaths we personally witness in the *Iliad* die in duels. These are the *promachoi*, the foremost warriors, champions who chose to fight out front, in the killing zone, where men either win glory or go down in death or both. It is less risky further back in the ranks, where one may go unseen and unchallenged by the enemy; but with safety comes nameless obscurity and insignificance, the fate of not being recognized at all, much less remembered. The battlefield of Troy is much like a dance floor, where you are a wallflower until you stand up and walk toward the other side of the room, find a worthy and attractive partner, and negotiate a dance. The difference between this and a dance, of course, is that only one of you walks away after the music stops. In a duel there are but two possibilities: kill or be killed. Either way you matter and are noticed. You provide a spectacle. In war as at a dance, those who sit it out have arguably neither lived nor died. It is as if they weren't even there. What we have called the "killing zone" may also be seen as a trysting place, because this is where warriors rendezvous for a "love-struggle, two bodies straining against each other in a match of death."[26] This was exactly how Homer saw and choreographed it, as a dance to the death, a dark mating of opposite forces, intimate and deadly, the "sweet rendezvous of war"

---

25. Marlantes, *What It Is Like*, 36.

26. Vermeule, *Aspects of Death*, 101.

(*polemou oaristus*).[27] Here, where men kill and die, we find ourselves in the bed of Ares and Aphrodite, where war and sex embrace.

To borrow an expression unknown to Homer but useful all the same to describe the ritual of battle on the killing fields of Troy, warriors "hook up" very much like lovers. They spy each other from a distance, sense interest, and draw closer, sometimes slowly, sometimes at whatever mad speed their legs or horses will convey them. Unless they have a past together, their ensuing "courtship" starts with words. Just as would-be lovers "sweet-talk" each other to provoke and measure their mutual attraction, so too would-be killers exchange insults and boasts to see what kind of rage they can ignite. It's too soon yet to make a move on the other. This is the time to dally, to engage in the fond, playful, increasingly familiar tête-à-tête (*oarismos*) of eager yet shy mates before going to bed and into each other's arms. The purpose of love talk is, of course, to incite desire, and here, on the field of death, it is also a matter of desire, the desire to kill, a confusing impulse unless impassioned with hatred and rage. "Violence," writes René Girard, "is always mingled with desire."[28] In keeping with the sexual ambiguity of these moments of preliminary intimacy, the words exchanged by enemies often aim to turn the other into a woman (or androgynous youth), weak and helpless before the might and designs of the man before her. Listen to this exchange and you will get the point:

> [Ajax to Hector:]
> Take a good look, Hector. This is what
> The heroes are like in the Greek army . . .
> But we still have a few good men to fight you.
> More than a few. It's your move.[29]

> [Hector to Ajax:]
> Telamonian Ajax . . .
> Don't try to unnerve me, as if I were
> Some kid, or a woman who wouldn't know
> One end of a spear from another.

27. Homer, *Iliad*, 17.228.
28. Girard, *Violence and the Sacred*, 145.
29. Homer, *Iliad*, 7.237–43.

I've been in a few battles and killed a few men,
And I know a few moves.[30]

These and numerous other comparable moments of battlefield "pillow talk" in the *Iliad* will make sharper sense to us if we set aside the distinction between "man" and "woman" and replace it with that between "lover" (*erastes*) and "beloved" (*eromenos*). The theory and practice of sex in ancient Greece are, in the main, androcentric, which is to say phallocentric and aggressively invasive. Sex was understood as a matter of penetration, and whatever the genders of the lovers, penetration meant power and the rest was weakness. There is no equality available in battle to the death, nor is there any such thing in love. To penetrate, then, was to exert power and to be penetrated was to accept weakness. These were the only two possibilities. Whether in love or in war, and regardless of the actual sex of the participants, to be penetrated was to play the woman, while to penetrate was to play the man. Replace the penis with a thrusting weapon, a spear or sword, and we move all but imperceptibly from the bed to the battlefield. Paris, we recall, in the *Iliad*, undergoes the reverse transition when he is wafted away, armor and all, from his duel-to-death with Menelaus to the love chamber of Helen. In the Greek imagination, battlefields and bedrooms adjoin each other, like connecting rooms in a hotel.

Eventually the time comes to move beyond words. In battle, this means that the warriors' *thumos* or battle fury is up and they draw closer. The foreplay of battle begins, and it is indeed "play" in that it is harmless—an inconsequential game or sport, provided it goes no further. But it does go further, as each tests the other's ferocity and skill. Now it's a matter of agility, skill, endurance, and opportunity. Each slashing blow, each wound, binds them together, as their blood mingles. They may find themselves in each other's arms, staring into each other's eyes, as they wrestle for dominance. When the moment comes, a thrust is made. If there is penetration, there is often an outcry, announcing great pain, and then a succumbing, as a dark mist glides in over the dying warrior to blow him out or away, like a flame or a feather.

It is much the same with lovers. When they see the light turn green, they leave talk behind and close in on each other, finding welcome ways of touching each other and of lingering where they want to. Sooner or later they too are wrestling in each other's arms, making their way to the moment

30. Ibid., 11.245–50.

of penetration and the excruciating scream of pleasure that follows. Soon, as if expiring, lovers collapse and drift off to sleep.

We have seen, then, that the rituals of love and war are much the same in Greek epic poetry: rendezvous, words of provocation, foreplay, struggle, consummation, and unconsciousness. Each ritual proceeds towards and culminates in a moment of erotic or deadly copulation, for which ancient Greek provides one word, *meignumi*, "joining," "mingling" or "mixing it up," used to denote both intercourse in battle and intercourse in bed. And lastly there is either sleep (*Hypnos*) or death (*Thanatos*)—twins in Greek mythology and all but indistinguishable in experience—to carry away warriors or lovers in their arms, gently, like a soft breeze. Thanatos, winged like his brother, is always portrayed as beautiful on the battlefield; for the warrior's death was seen by the Greeks as a beautiful death, a happy death, like death in the arms of a lover: "When a young man is killed in war, / Even though his body is slashed with bronze, / He lies there beautiful in death, noble."[31] This from no less than Priam, anticipating the death of his own son.

To bring to a close this chapter and its exploration of the entanglement of love and war in the ancient Greek imagination, we will focus on surely one of the most poignant and heart-rending scenes in the *Iliad*, a moment when the rituals of sex and battle nearly exchange places. It is a moment of sheer desperation for the Trojan forces and for their loved ones who watch them from the city walls. The army, routed and in full retreat, floods through the city's gates to the temporary refuge offered by its walls. All but Hector.

> Outside, the Greeks
> Formed up close to the wall, locking their shields.
> In the dead air between the Greeks
> And Troy's Western Gate, Destiny
> Had Hector pinned, waiting for death.[32]

Achilles, "a single point of light on Troy's dusty plain,"[33] races toward Hector to claim his life and Hector awaits him. It will be a colossal duel to the death, a battle dance like no other. From above, on the walls, Hector's mother and father plead with him to come inside and live to fight another

31. Ibid., 22.79–82.
32. Ibid., 22.5–9.
33. Ibid., 22.32.

day, to no avail. Hector holds his ground and resolves to meet Achilles man to man, either killing him or dying in the effort.

But for one brief moment a crack appears in his resolve and he wonders about laying down his weapons and making a deal with Achilles, to give back Helen and everything else Paris took from Menelaus a decade earlier, to turn back time and call an end to the killing. Then, in the next instant, with Achilles bearing down on him, Hector knows these thoughts for what they are—sheer fantasy. He is going into battle. Yes, but even as he does, he imagines himself not a warrior but a lover, not the hated enemy (*ekhthros*) of Achilles, but his beloved (*eromenos*).

> But why am I talking to myself like this?
> I can't go out there unarmed. Achilles
> Will cut me down in cold blood if I take off
> My armor and go out to meet him
> Naked like a woman. This is no time
> For talking, the way a boy and a girl
> Whisper to each other from oak tree or rock,
> A boy and a girl with all their sweet talk.
> Better to lock up in mortal combat
> As soon as possible and see to whom
> God on Olympus grants the victory.[34]

This last conversation of Hector with himself is not so much a wish as it is a prophecy. Soon after, he runs for his life around the walls of Troy, only to turn and face his killer straight on. Hector will lie beneath these same walls and become the naked woman he has already imagined. Then, after Achilles pulls out the spear with which he just penetrated the body of Hector, he strips the body and his fellow Greek warriors collect around the corpse.

> The other Greeks crowded around
> And could not help but admire Hector's
> Beautiful body, but still they stood there
> Stabbing their spears into him, smirking.
> "Hector's a lot softer to the touch now
> Than he was when he was burning our ships."[35]

34. Ibid., 22.138–48.
35. Ibid., 22.409–14.

The scene has turned sexual, even pornographic. A clean combat kill has become gang rape. Hatred has turned to desire, a violent and dark desire, to penetrate the soft, limp, yielding flesh of a beautiful youth. War, it has been said, is necrophilia, and it is difficult to dispute that claim from where we stand at this moment.

3

Killing

Moral Agency and Pollution

IN THE LAST CHAPTER we revealed and reflected on the entanglement of love and war in the ancient Greek imagination. This curious and counterintuitive fusion of lovemaking and warmaking will endure into the Christian era and prove critical in the church's earliest deliberations and decrees regarding the moral precariousness of marriage and military service. With that piece of our narrative in place, then, it is time now to turn to another set of considerations equally critical to the unfolding story and eventual argument of this book. What I have in mind is the surprisingly complex question of just how responsible we are—or are not—for our actions, say for example our actions of copulating and killing. Once again, we find our precedent and paradigm in Greek tragedy, this time in the famed and familiar figure of Oedipus, in whose complex, or at least complexity, we all have our own share.

In antiquity, there were a number of versions of or takes on the Oedipus legend, but for the moment we will confine ourselves to the one we find in Sophocles' *Oedipus the King* (more accurately translated "Oedipus the Tyrant"). In this drama, the city of Thebes is in full crisis, afflicted with a deadly plague brought down on the entire population by the misdeeds of just one of Thebes' citizens, a man guilty of murder and incest, who has yet to be found out and punished. This man brings pollution (*miasma*) to all, for pollution, like the plague, is wildly contagious. Oedipus, as yet clueless to the identity of the polluting agent, takes it on himself as king to track down the perpetrator and to make him pay for his crimes. What he doesn't know but soon finds out is that he is both the tracker and the tracked, the judge and the judged. Once revealed to himself as the killer of his own father, the lover of his own mother, and the brother of his own offspring, his self-inflicted justice is swift. He pierces his own eyes and casts himself from the throne into permanent banishment. He will spend the rest of his days homeless on the wild slopes of Mount Parnassus, where he had spent his first days of life as an infant, tethered to a rock and left as prey.

For Oedipus there would seem to have been little doubt that he was responsible for having killed his father and bedded his mother. The evidence that he had done both was incontrovertible, and so he and no one else was the living pollutant cursing his own city to undeserved agony. He acted without hesitation to remove himself from the sight of others and to deny himself even the light of day. For the audience of this drama, however, the case may not be so easily or clearly closed. Not having paid the same price as had the citizens of Thebes for the crimes of Oedipus, they and we may experience pity and even sympathy for this man, who for all he knew killed a stranger in self-defense and married a young widow out of mutual desire. As the story of this ill-starred man spills out on stage, we see that he consistently acted in the dark, nearly as blind with eyes as he later became without any. No matter how lucidly he sought to steer a straight course, he acted in consistent ignorance of what he was actually doing. Surely, he never wanted to shed his father's blood, much less spill his own seed where a son does not belong. But he did both, by accident, as it were. He sums up the truth of his life thus far when he says that he is the child of chance, which is to say that his life is and always has been beyond his ken, out of his control. He has acted and his actions have had their inevitable consequences, but in all of this he has never known what he was doing.

The question here, for us if not for Oedipus, is whether anyone should be held accountable for deeds done in ignorance and without intent. Sophocles seems to come down, in this drama, on the side of full accountability. In other ancient versions of the story, Oedipus neither blinded nor banished himself, but continued on as ruling king of Thebes after he had learned the truth and consequences of what he had done. Sophocles may have been the first to condemn him to sightless exile. In doing so, he looked to the consequences of Oedipus' actions. There was, after all, a dead father and king, and a queen mother who hanged herself in shame when she learned that she had shared a bed with her son, and four children whose father was at the same time their brother. All this was the debris left by Oedipus' deeds, witting or unwitting, willing or unwilling. It would seem that at the main gate of Thebes there might have hung a sign, like one frequently found in ceramic shops, that reads, "You broke it, you bought it." Such signs and the policies behind them refuse to take into account that most items broken in shops are broken by chance or accident. Why? Because a pot shattered by accident is no less shattered than one broken on purpose. Someone has to pay for it, and who else but the person whose action caused it to fall? It is one thing for me not to know what I am doing and quite another for me not to know what I have done. Actions, it seems, are to be defined by their consequences, which unlike the actor's awareness or intent are at the end of the day plain for all to see.

Whatever we make of Sophocles' harsh treatment of Oedipus in *Oedipus the King*, we need to revisit and revise the case against Oedipus, as did Sophocles himself, nearly four decades later, in a play all but written with his last breaths and produced in the year following his death. *Oedipus at Colonus* brings both the life of Sophocles and the life of Oedipus to a stunning close. To borrow an image from the text, the playwright and his protagonist have come to the final lap of life's long course and are rounding its last turning-post. Both have grown wiser or, at the least, have changed their minds about the tragedy played out ever so many years earlier. Oedipus returns to Athens or, more precisely, to the Athenian "suburb" of Colonus (the birthplace of Sophocles), in his own words no longer to bring a curse but rather to bestow blessings. Of those blessings the first is clear-sighted speech, a boon not commonly at the disposal of a blind man. All Oedipus asks in return is a resting place, a final resting place to be more exact. Unfortunately, the place he chooses happens to be a *temenos* or sacred enclosure belonging to the formidable and fierce Daughters of Darkness and of the Goddess Earth, and he is far from welcome there. It is holy ground, and he remains, in the all-cleansing keepers' eyes, a notorious pollutant, defiled and defiling. In his own eyes, however, he is now innocent, without guilt and without stain.

There, in the holy grove of the Daughters of Darkness, Oedipus sheds fresh light on his past deeds and pleads a case that, to all appearances, had not previously occurred to him or to Sophocles. He asks how anyone could accuse him of being innately evil, evil in his nature, his core, when the wrong he did was unwitting and unintended. No one is made evil by unwilling deeds done in ignorance. In fact, he argues, it is more true to say that he suffered those deeds than to say that he did them. Oedipus the perpetrator has become Oedipus the victim. When the Daughters of Darkness object and remind him of the irrefutable fact that he has his father's blood on his hands, he in turn reminds them of another irrefutable fact—that he killed in ignorance—and this means that he is innocent before the law. The word he uses here is *katharos*, "spotless." But is innocence before the law the same as innocence before the gods? Even if Oedipus cannot be convicted in a court of men and must go free on a technicality or extenuation, will not his pollution, his stain, still cling to him for the rest of his days? Apparently not. So far from his being abhorrent to the gods, Sophocles describes how the gods, impatient for Oedipus to join them, take him directly to themselves, sparing him the agony of death.

How can we grasp or explain this transformation of Oedipus from pariah to godsend? One clue may lie in his suffering. Before he was blessed he was broken, utterly. And with suffering, we are often told, comes cleansing and transformation. Of what Oedipus endured in his unthinkably harsh and endless exile, we are told only this:

> Think of some shore in the north
> Concussive waves make stream
> This way and that in the gales of winter:
> It is like that with him:
> The wild wrack breaking over him
> From head to foot, and coming on forever;
> Now from the plunging down of the sun,
> Now from the sunrise quarter,
> Now from where the noonday gleams,
> Now from the light and the north.[1]

We know well the power of nature, left to its own resources, to cleanse itself of all but the most toxic pollutants. Perhaps nature has a similar power over its most wondrous yet wayward children, the broken race of men and women, to make them new again. Many claim to have experienced as much, and Sophocles (on behalf of Oedipus) seems to have been one of them.

Regardless of where Sophocles finally came down on the matter of Oedipus' guilt or innocence, we are left by these plays with two very

1. Sophocles, *Oedipus at Colonus*, 1240–48.

different and clearly conflicting understandings of human action. In the first case, action is defined by its consequences, and in the second case, action is defined by its intent. Both understandings have a certain common sense on their side. If I have done something that cannot be undone, am I really entitled to claim that I didn't do it just because at the time I didn't know what I was doing? Does it make no difference or does it make all the difference that I didn't mean to do it? The house I burned down by accident remains in ashes. The child I ran down because I didn't see her still lies dead. These were not "acts of god." They were acts of mine. At the same time, how can I be held accountable for what I never consciously or willingly chose to do? What if I chose to smoke in bed or to drive while intoxicated, but never chose to destroy a house or a life? Am I an arsonist or a murderer simply because I have a weakness, simply because I lit a last cigarette or took an extra drink? And what about in war? What if I shot the wrong person, shelled the wrong house, bombed the wrong target? Do I have innocent blood on my hands? It seems we cannot easily or perhaps ever leave behind either of these ways of defining action nor the questions they raise. Rather, they will follow us every step of our way through this book and beyond, as they should; for there is truth in both. Taken alone, either one misses the complex reality of human agency.

It may be that the urgency of these matters will fail to strike us until we move from ancient tragedy to modern tragedy, from the Athenian stage to today's news. One example, I believe, is all that it will take to convince us that Oedipus is not alone in his bewilderment and shame over actions he never intended and yet is helpless to deny or undo. The example I have in mind is a "crime" that for all its unimaginable horror happens frequently enough to have been given its own unique name: "forgotten baby syndrome." This is when an infant or toddler is inadvertently left locked in a car and dies of hyperthermia before anyone notices, and it happens more often than anyone would care to imagine. In the United States, since 1998, an average of thirty-eight children per year have died of vehicular heat stroke, which comes to one death every 9.6 days.[2] In well over half of these cases, the adult responsible for leaving and locking the child in the car was unaware of having done so—a simple matter of inadvertence, preoccupation, forgetfulness, or multitasking, at least until we focus on the victim, the dead child. Then it looks more like murder, which would account for the fact that in roughly 60 percent of such deaths, the parents or guardians responsible

2. These and other related data and statistics may be found at www.kidsandcars.org.

face felony charges. While there are isolated instances of the conscious, deliberate abandonment of children in overheated vehicles, in most cases the offending parent acts without any awareness, much less intent. Who would claim or imagine otherwise? All the same, we may wonder, who does such a thing? Relying on case studies, we would have to answer: doctors, teachers, clergy, nurses, soldiers, police officers, the neighbor next door—anyone sufficiently stressed, exhausted, or distracted to forget for a moment that a child's life is at stake. A moment ago in this discussion, I asked whether conscious intent makes all the difference or no difference at all when we act. Apparently, when the act is that of locking an infant in an overheated car it makes very little difference in many people's eyes. Weighed against a dead child, who cares about intent? Often not even the mother or father whose child it is, or was; for they are often their own harshest judges, and must be protected against themselves and their own merciless self-rage.

Since it is easier to walk past statistics than it is to forget stories, we may do well to consider here the accounts of several parents who, like Oedipus, unwittingly did the unthinkable. On the morning of June 17, 2011, in Bristow, Virginia, Karen Murphy, a forty-year-old mother and veterinarian, drove to her place of employment, the Caring Hands Animal Clinic, and after a day's work drove home and parked her Honda Odyssey minivan in the driveway. Then her husband called her, saying that he had gone to the day-care center to pick up their two-year-old son Ryan and that he was not there. It was only then that Karen Murphy discovered her son dead in his car seat. Her screams, it was reported, could be heard for blocks. On July 5, 2011, Karen Murphy was indicted by a grand jury on one count of felony murder and one count of felony child neglect. Her case was complicated by the fact that she had left her son in the minivan six months earlier but soon realized her error and rescued him before any harm was done.[3]

On an otherwise routine summer day in 2003, Mark Warschauer, a professor of education at the University of California at Irvine, walked to lunch and then back toward his office.[4] Seeing a crowd in the parking lot, he drew closer and realized that his car was the center of the crowd's attention. The police had shattered his window and removed his dead ten-month-old son. This was his first reminder all day that he had forgotten to leave off his boy at day care, and it came too late. He was not charged with a

3. See White, "Prince William Mother Charged."
4. This account and that of Raelyn Balfour are taken from Gene Weingarten's Pulitzer Prize–winning article "Fatal Distraction: Forgetting a Child in the Backseat of a Car."

crime, but he contemplated suicide. Army reservist and combat veteran Raelyn Balfour, another parent who fell prey to one too many coincidences and distractions and left her child to die, is more accepting of herself. "I don't feel I need to forgive myself," she says plainly, "because what I did was not intentional." The local prosecutor was less understanding, and she was charged with second-degree murder, with a possible forty-year prison sentence. Her jury, on the other hand, delivered a unanimous not guilty verdict. The jury foreman called it "a big doggone accident" and another jury member said it was "an honest mistake." Responses to these and other similar cases recorded in the media range from expressions of profound sympathy to calls for the death sentence.

It could happen to anyone. This is what the evidence suggests and what simple honesty nudges us to admit. Oedipus said as much regarding his own misfortune when he said that it was truer to say that he suffered his actions than to say that he did them. Claiming that our actions "happen" to us, however, seems a stretch. With a dead child in the backseat, our first impulse is not to see the perfectly healthy but forgetful parent as the victim, however bereaved and despairing he or she may be.

But what about a homicide in which the slayer and the slain are both small children, in fact identical twins? Now I have in mind a tragedy that I shall never be able to forget, as it happened to a young family I once knew. I will tell the story as it was told to me. The four of them—two parents and two boys, maybe six years of age at the time—came home from the movies on an unexceptional Saturday afternoon after having seen a swashbuckling adventure film of some sort, perhaps *Peter Pan*. The parents were resting before dinner and the two boys had gone downstairs to the family room to play, on fire to choose their parts and reenact their favorite sword-fighting scenes from the movie. After waving first their arms and then rolled-up newspapers at one another for a while, they stole up to the kitchen, fetched two more realistic blades from the knife rack, and descended to the play-room to resume battle. They had of course been told countless times never to go near knives (much less wield them at each other), but fantasy and excitement can wipe all that away. After minutes of harmless melée, it happened. One boy stretched out his blade at the very moment when the other boy, perched on a couch cushion, lost his balance and fell forward. The knife pierced his chest and heart and he bled to death on the carpet at the feet of his twin.

An accident? Of course. Intended? Of course not. Anyone's fault? Yes, but the fault pales before its consequence. Every household kitchen has knives, and knives unlike guns are not usually kept under lock and key. The boys were careless and disobedient, but they were also mere children. No one meant this to happen, but that was little consolation to anyone. After months of trying to cope, the family moved away, far away. No one blamed them. Everyone pitied them. Then why did they leave? Why did they go into exile? Maybe for the same reason that Oedipus did.

By now in our discussion surely we have been struck with the confusing complexity of human agency and accountability, particularly when we confront and consider acts that may be considered criminal, sinful, or shameful. It may be helpful to think of all of these acts as "violations" and then to sort them out, as best we can, according to what line, as it were, has in each instance been trespassed. Some actions violate "the law" or civil legislation and so are judged to be "illegal," while others violate "morality," a more elusive norm grounded in either religion or reason or both. The most universal of all moral codes is the simple prescription known as the Golden Rule, which enjoins us to act toward others as we would have them act toward us. One of the earliest and most inevitable disillusionments or scandals in life comes with the realization that a sizeable gulf separates "the legal" from "the moral" or "the just." The law all too often, as Plato realized millennia ago, represents no more than the legislated self-interest of the powerful, and the powerful are rarely known for their moral vision or conduct. On the other hand, those who are most committed to leading moral lives can and do at times find themselves compelled to break the law. This fact complicates the concept of "crime." Capital punishment, for example, is legal in some states and illegal in others. What is lawful in Texas is murder in Minnesota, which fact says nothing about the morality of the death penalty. Likewise, killing in war is sanctioned by the state, provided that the war is in Afghanistan and not in Chicago. Armies are legal and gangs are not. But none of this fully explains why so many returning veterans, like Noah Pierce, are consumed with guilt and shame for the killing they have done, or why a mother who forgot her infant in the backseat of a car cannot forgive herself, or why a small child with his brother's blood on his hands must go into exile.

There must be another category of crime that is independent of civil laws and moral codes, crime that anyone can commit without awareness or intent, crime that can just "happen" to you. This, quite tentatively, we will call "metaphysical crime" for lack of a better term. In ancient Greece and many other early cultures, such an act would bring with it the burden of pollution (*miasma*), calling for a period of isolation as well as one or other ritual of purification (*katharsis*). Such ideas and rituals, of course, are so far from current belief and fashion that we moderns and postmoderns mostly regard them as primitive and superstitious, which may be one reason why our minds fall blank on the fact that some remote forests of New England and the Pacific Northwest are to this day, more than thirty-five years after the Vietnam War ended, still inhabited by small bands of vets who have lived out their postwar lives in self-imposed woodland exile, though some are beginning now in their old age to seek services and assistance from the nearest VA facility or Vet Center. Like Oedipus, in the final lap of life's long race, they need and seek a place to rest.

Pollution is a vast topic, not only within classical studies but also within the much more extensive reach of anthropology. There is no question of our coming to an inclusive or conclusive understanding or account here of this at once archaic and abiding phenomenon. It will be enough for us to glimpse its reality, its rough form, and its disturbing force. *Miasma*, the ancient Greek version of pollution, encompasses such sweeping categories or concepts as defilement, disfigurement, impurity, sin, and accursedness. Pollution refers to a contaminated state or condition in which the polluted one is both endangered and dangerous, as if infected with a contagious disease. Such a one, while at risk personally, at the same time represents a risk to others. Critical for our purposes here is the fact that pollution does not imply any conscious or willful culpability. Rather, "it is the automatic consequence of an action, belongs to the world of external events, and operates with the same ruthless indifference to motive as a typhoid germ."[5] While pollution may well be accompanied by moral guilt or legal liability, it need not be. It can happen to anyone—someone in the wrong place at the wrong time, someone who inadvertently, or for good reason, or for no reason at all, commits a polluting act, such as homicide.

Killing may be unwitting, accidental, sanctioned, or forbidden. Either way, there is pollution. Blood clings to the hands of anyone who sheds it. The purification of killers in nearly every instance requires among other things a period of exile.[6] The duration of such exile in ancient Greece would

5. Dodds, *Greeks and the Irrational*, 36.

6. An exception to this rule is the warrior. In Athens and apparently throughout ancient Greece, killing in battle seems not to have carried the same pollution as other

reasonably vary according to the severity of the homicidal offense and the degree of legal and moral culpability assigned to the killer. What's more, the necessity of exile or expulsion could extend even beyond the human sphere. "In Athens, animals or inanimate objects that had caused death were tried in the Prytaneum and, if found guilty, expelled beyond the boundaries of Attica."[7] But what of someone who has brought about the death of another with clear, methodic intent but without lifting a finger, much less shedding blood? I have in mind anyone who has someone else do his killing for him, a killer for hire. Is the "employer" or only the assassin polluted in such an instance? In the *Laws*, Plato is clear on this. While the assassin quite literally has blood on his hands, the other, the one who "purposed the death of another and brought him to his end by death and contrivance," is nonetheless polluted and bears "the stain of homicide on his soul."[8] A similar point can be and has been made today regarding the responsibility of those in power who send others to kill in their name or in advancement of their policies. "I do not doubt," writes Karl Marlantes,

> that most of our leaders take their responsibilities very seriously, but only if they see that *they* are actually doing the killing can they make a more conscious decision. Ideally, they should know ahead of time that *they* will have to face nightmares the rest of their lives over the killing. It will make for better decisions.[9]

In war, the men in the front ranks, it has often been said, are only the tip of the spear, the point that draws blood, while those who send them off to war hold the spear firmly in their hands when it does its killing. They are bloodless but not without stain.

In any kind of killing there is blood on the killer's hands that must be washed off. Those bloodied by their deeds are not only to be excluded from sacred spaces but from the city itself, the everyday community of men and women. But it is not only blood shed in anger that is dangerous and suspect; menses and afterbirth also signal pollution and a prescribed period of

---

killing. Though there may well have been special rites of purification for returning warriors, there is no evidence of their being required to endure any period of isolation or exile. When we consider that military service was required of every adult male citizen until the age of sixty, it stands to reason that returning warriors would not be sent into exile. To do so would be to reduce the male population to children and old men.

7. Parker, *Miasma*, 117.

8. Plato, *Laws* 872a.

9. Marlantes, *What It Is Like*, 127.

ritual quarantine. Seminal discharge too is not without its risks and consequences. Once again we find that sex and violence share the same, or at the
least adjoining, semiotic space. And is this surprising? It may not require
too great a stretch for us, even today in an often stubbornly secular world,
to grant that the giving or taking of life are serious, even sacred, matters,
set apart from our more mundane, relatively inconsequential, everyday
occupations, the ones we forget as fast as we do them. Shopping, texting,
surfing the Net, or watching TV, for example, are not "liminal" activities,
requiring us to cross a metaphysically fraught border and to enter a realm
that does not admit of easy return. Making love, life, war, or death is not,
we know, like making dinner. Unlike meal preparation, these acts alter and
thus alienate or estrange us. They set us apart. It may be that ancient beliefs
and rituals of pollution, exile, and purification arose from this realization
and provided a path back to the circle of human fellowship for those who
found themselves suddenly outside it.

In the ancient world there were many traditional agents and rituals of
purification or healing for those who found themselves polluted by what
they had done or by what they had experienced. Water and fire were both
employed to cleanse and remove contamination or stain. A less ritual and
arguably more real path to purification was often found in suffering and
endurance. This may take the form of what we often call "penance" and
involve pain, denial, or hardship, such as fasting, sleeplessness, poverty, ex-
posure, or pilgrimage. We have already seen that these are precisely the elements of Oedipus' purgation in *Oedipus at Colonus,* wherein he is likened
to "some shore in the north / Concussive waves make stream / This way and
that in the gales of winter." The most powerful and effective of all purifying
agents, however, may well have been and may still be the passage of time.
That time heals where all else fails is a well-weathered truism, which admittedly makes it neither true nor false. But in the case of Oedipus the passage
of time surely did him no harm. Rather, it transfigured him from outcast to
prophet, from scapegoat to a kind of saint.

Looking back over this brief survey and discussion of guilt and shame,
I have distinguished legal guilt from moral guilt and both from pollution or
shame, which is not to deny that in practice all three may well overlap and
become entangled. The most crucial distinction here may be that between
guilt and shame, both of which today haunt and torment many if not most
combat veterans. In fact, actions that provoke either guilt or shame or both
are likely the source of the most profound trauma experienced in war. These
include perpetrating, failing to prevent, or even merely witnessing acts that

violate our most deeply held moral or religious convictions. These actions may not and need not include what we ordinarily consider to be war crimes or atrocities. After all, acts that are routine in war, such as the hunting and killing of others like ourselves, are clearly criminal outside of war. When we add cruelty and chance to the mix and realize that the killing of children like our children and old men and women like our fathers and mothers and women like our wives and lovers are also common if not routine in war, then it is little wonder that those responsible may find themselves defiled and in need of cleansing, regardless of whether the blood on them was shed by accident, unwittingly, under orders, or in a moment of blind rage.

In any triage of war's invisible wounds, guilt presents a less lethal threat to sanity and survival than does shame. In a declared war, guilt before the law is rarely an issue, and moral guilt, while it may well cause grievous inner distress and pain, is likely to be self-contained. A soul afflicted with guilt is not thereby a threat to others. Guilt is not contagious. Instead, it is most often suffered in private and healed, if at all, outside the public eye, through such means as memory, narrative, confession, and reparations. Shame is another matter, involving a global or comprehensive devaluation of the self and a consequent inner compulsion to withdraw from others, especially those others who are nearest and dearest. Guilt carries the weight of having done something evil, whereas shame's burden is that of having become evil, to the core. It is one thing to have done something abhorrent and unforgivable, and another to be abhorrent and unforgivable. Guilt, once acknowledged and addressed, often evokes understanding and compassion from others, and this initial bond can be the beginning of one's return to inner peace. Shame, on the other hand, anticipates or even invites rejection by others and leads the way to ever deeper and more extensive withdrawal for the sake of self and others. In this and other ways, shame mirrors pollution, which suggests that the shame experienced by many veterans today might well be given the diagnosis of "pollution" as the ancients understood it. Indeed, many veterans, consumed with irrational and seemingly incurable shame, act plague-ridden, their souls sick unto death, convinced that their dark malaise is contagious and that they themselves, no longer worthy of care, are a danger to everyone they love and to everyone who loves them.

Not everyone in the ancient world, however, gave any credence or quarter to pollution. Among the classical Greeks, Euripides stands out as one who denied its reality and power. We find a striking instance of this dismissal in his *Suppliant Women,* a play about the horrifying aftermath of fratricidal war. His focus is on the senseless suffering of those who neither provoked nor pursued the war, the citizens of Thebes, the survivors. Like so many of his plays, *The Suppliant Women* is essentially a plea for humanity, even and especially in war. The moment in the play that I would highlight here is when the Messenger relates how Theseus, the king of Athens, attended to the dead left to rot on the battlefield. He is described as having washed the corpses with his own hands, an act that surely polluted him. When asked how the king could have taken on himself such a burden of shame, the Messenger asks, in return, how it is that sharing in our common evils and ills can possibly be shameful (i.e., polluting).[10] We cannot allow, as Euripides sees it, the human circle to be broken.

Surely the most poignant expression of Euripides' characteristic disregard for pollution and shame is to be found in the *Herakles*. Once again it is Theseus who embodies the compassion and courage required to ignore the dangers of contagion and curse posed by bloodshed and atrocity. When Theseus makes his entrance in this tragedy, Herakles has already slaughtered his own wife and children in a fit of hallucinatory madness brought down on him by powers beyond his consciousness or control. Although he did not know what he was doing when he murdered his family, he knows only too well now what he has done. In shame and despair, he lies prostrate on the ground and covers his head with his cloak. He wants neither to be seen nor to live. Withdrawal from the sight of men and from life itself is all that he now hopes and longs for. Theseus has something else in mind for his friend and offers his hand. What follows is one of the most transcendent scenes in all of Greek drama.

> HERAKLES: Theseus, did you witness the battle I waged against my own children?
> THESEUS: I've been told of it.
> And what you point to tells me the rest.
> HERAKLES: Why have you exposed my head to the sun?
> THESEUS: You are a mortal, a human being.
> You cannot pollute what belongs to the gods.
> HERAKLES: Poor man, leave, get away from here!
> I am unholy, defiled, polluted.
> THESEUS: The demon of pollution cannot pass from friend to friend . . .
>
> THESEUS: Enough tears, poor man. Now, up on your feet.
> HERAKLES: I can't. My legs don't any longer bear my weight.

10. See *The Suppliant Women*, line 768.

THESEUS: Misfortune does that, even to the strong.
It pulls them down.
HERAKLES: If only I could become a rock,
unfeeling, oblivious of evil.
THESEUS: Stop that. Just give me your hand.
I'm your friend, and I'm here to help you.
HERAKLES: I'm covered with blood. It will stain your robe.
THESEUS: Let it all wipe off on me. Don't let that hold you back.
I'm not leaving without you.[11]

Theseus insists on this—there is no such thing as pollution among friends. And Euripides, throughout the corpus of his writings, makes clear that the natural or "default" relationship, as it were, between human beings is that of friendship. Anything less is failure.

To conclude this discussion of human agency and responsibility, we turn briefly now to a more radical understanding of human action and accountability and a more sweeping dismissal of contagious pollution than any we have encountered so far. Both are to be found in the gospels of the Christian New Testament and so are believed by Christians to be the authentic teachings of Jesus Christ. Given the focus and trajectory of this text, it should be obvious that these teachings will prove foundational for all that follows, which is not to say that they will prove immune to challenge and criticism.

No one who reads the Christian Scriptures can fail to note that Jesus is far more concerned with the inner state and disposition of the soul or heart than with the outer observance of the law. Sin is a state or condition before it is an act. It lies hidden before it becomes manifest or visible—hidden from others but not from God, from whom nothing is hidden, much less the hearts of men. The act of sin is done first in the heart (*kardía*) before it is done (if at all) outwardly, in the flesh, before the eyes of others.

> You have heard that it was said to those of ancient times, "You shall not murder"; and "whoever murders shall be liable to judgment." But I say to you that if you are angry with a brother or sister, you will be liable to judgment . . .
>
> You have heard that it was said, "You shall not commit adultery." But I say to you that everyone who looks at a woman with lust has already committed adultery with her in his heart. (Matt 5:21–22, 27–28)

11. Euripides in *Herakles*, lines 1231–34 and 1394–1400.

These words of Jesus make it clear that actions are to be defined not so much by their consequences as by their intent. If I am a murderer in my heart then it matters little whether I have any corpses to show for it; and if I murder unwittingly or unwillingly or without murder in my heart, the fact that I have blood on my hands does not mean that my heart is not pure.

And what if I am guilty of murder or adultery in the eyes of God? What hope is there for forgiveness? What manner and duration of exile, what ritual of purification, am I required to observe? In the New Testament, sinners are to confess their sins, turn to God, and seek forgiveness like children from a loving father. Jesus forgives sin as easily as one might forgive a debt, expecting at the same time that his forgiveness will be remembered and imitated. But turning to sin is a more profound misstep than slipping into debt. The state of sin is more like death than indebtedness, and the remission of sins is more like raising the dead than clearing the ledger. In the New Testament there is little attention paid to any legal or moral codes or to crimes that violate them. Criminals and reprobates find themselves welcome at the table of the Lord, so long as they turn wholeheartedly to him in belief and love. "Blessed are the pure in heart," assures Jesus, "for they will see God" (Matt 5:8).

In contrast with the generally scrupulous concern for ritual purity found in ancient Greece and Israel, Jesus displayed remarkable, even shocking disregard for the laws of pollution that he as a Jew should have observed. He walked freely amidst, touched, and healed those afflicted with every manner of physical affliction, deformity, and decay, even (in the case of Lazarus) entering the tomb of a rotting corpse. Demons or unclean spirits, too, posed no threat to him. Still less did he fear adulterers or prostitutes, soldiers or tax collectors. Ironically, it was a relatively trivial matter that prompted Jesus to set out quite fully and plainly his views on pollution and sin. One day the Pharisees and scribes, those brittle embodiments of ritual righteousness, accosted Jesus over the fact that his disciples were in the practice of eating with unwashed hands. This was all the opportunity he needed to gather a crowd and to teach them a crucial lesson. "Listen and understand," he said,

> It is not what goes into the mouth that defiles a person, but it is what comes out of the mouth that defiles. . . . Do you not see that whatever goes into the mouth enters the stomach, and goes out into the sewer? But what comes out of the mouth proceeds from the heart, and this is what defiles. For out of the heart come

> evil intentions, murder, adultery, fornication, theft, false witness, slander. These are what defile a person, but to eat with unwashed hands does not defile. (Matt 15:10, 17–20)

Sin and pollution are matters of the heart, not of the hands; and matters of the heart lie hidden to all but the eyes of God. Only God is able to judge, to sort the clean from the unclean. Only this can explain the startling words of intercession spoken by the crucified Jesus on behalf of his tormentors: "Father, forgive them; for they do not know what they are doing" (Luke 23:34).[12] After all, these are no ordinary murderers. In the eyes of Christians they are the murderers of God. If the consequence of an action were ever to be allowed to eclipse intent, this would seem to be the occasion to do so. Given the incalculable magnitude of the crime, why would anyone care to measure the awareness of the perpetrators? But Jesus has been clear on this. For something to "come out of the mouth" and "proceed from the heart" there must be full awareness and will, and these men, the soldiers who nailed Jesus to his cross, did not know fully what they were doing. For this reason they are to be forgiven.

These words bring us to a new place, a new conception of agency and responsibility that will profoundly reshape the discussion of war and sex, killing and lovemaking, bloodshed and propagation in the early Christian centuries and clear down to the present day. The urgent question posed by Neoptolemus—"Is there no place, then, for repentance?"—has received an unexpected answer. Forgiveness, even spiritual rebirth, are at hand. But are they even necessary? After all, who can ever say that he—any more than did Oedipus in Thebes—really knows what he is doing or what he has done? Are not our hearts hidden even from ourselves, or perhaps most from ourselves? If all sin, even the murder of God, can be forgiven, does this signal a new opportunity for innocence or a new path to impunity? Pollution was a terrible prospect for anyone on his way to take a life, but it may be that purity of heart will prove still more dangerous. Christianity brought no end to war, much less to sex, but it did raise a novel question: can a Christian go to battle or to bed without sin?

12. The authenticity of this verse has been questioned on the grounds that it does not appear in every surviving early gospel manuscript, but that fact alone would seem insufficient grounds for singling it out for dismissal.

4

Imperial Rome

Warriors and Believers

"Go THEREFORE AND MAKE disciples of all nations, baptizing them in the name of the Father and of the Son and of the Holy Spirit, and teaching them everything that I have commanded you. And remember I am with you always, to the end of the age" (Matt 28:19–20). In two of the gospels—Matthew and Mark—this mission call to preach the *evangelion* or "good news" to the furthest reaches of the peopled world comprised the last words of Jesus to the chosen eleven, his last will and testament, as it were. Whether the historical Jesus ever spoke these words to his disciples will remain forever a matter of dispute. Even so, there is no disputing the fact that in the ensuing decades and centuries they and their successors endeavored to do exactly what these words enjoined them to do. The sticking point from the start and to the present day, however, is that even the eleven, much less the countless millions who followed them, were never quite able to reach agreement on exactly what Jesus had taught them or what he had otherwise commanded them to do. Here, keeping to the focus of this book, we are concerned with only two curiously entangled areas of such instruction and command, the one having to do with sex and the other having to do with war. The relevant questions considered and debated by the first Christians were—simply stated—whether marriage and military service are compatible with the teachings of Jesus and the Christian life. The sinfulness of adultery, fornication, and murder was never seriously in doubt in Christian circles.

The injunction of Jesus to "go therefore and make disciples of all nations" may evoke and be compared with the much earlier, to say the least, marching order given to Adam and Eve to "be fruitful and multiply, and fill the earth and subdue it" (Gen 1:28). One eventual and memorable outcome of Adam and Eve's filling the earth with progeny was the Tower of Babel, an icon of mass confusion between peoples and of their endemic waywardness in the eyes of the Creator. And how could it have been otherwise? At the end of the day, multiplicity and diversity are often two words for the same thing, particularly where religion is concerned. So too, when the eleven, in their distinct missions, proved fruitful and indeed multiplied, filling the earth with disciples, they also inevitably sowed seeds of confusion. The fact that baptism was and is seen as a second birth renders the carnal fertility of the world's first parents an especially suitable foreshadowing of the spiritual fertility of Christianity's first preachers. With great numbers came great disagreement. The historical Jesus presumably spoke with one voice, but those who spoke for him in the future spoke with many tongues, in many tongues, and found it all but impossible to say the same thing.

The elephant in the room, or more accurately in the church, from the start was the gap or gulf between Jesus and Christianity, and it is a gap that has only widened with time. Gandhi, a latecomer and outsider for sure, is said to have once remarked that "I like your Christ, I do not like your Christians. Your Christians are so unlike your Christ." But insiders too have said as much, asking themselves and others for millennia whether Jesus was or would ever care to be a Christian. Paul of Tarsus, Saint Paul, grandfathered into the circle of the apostles, is often credited with or accused of being the actual founder of Christianity. Then, too, in our search for first roots, there were the church fathers, "founding fathers" as some see them, whose voices—at least as far as we can tell—dominated the deliberations of the early Christian church; but their legacy is lessened by the fact that they silenced their foes and quarreled among themselves. And what, we might ask, about the church mothers, such as Marcella and Paula, two Christian widows mentored by Saint Jerome, who were among the most skilled and learned theological scholars of the early church?[1] While admired and

1. In the taxonomy of sainthood, there were only three traditional categories: martyr, virgin, and confessor, and the third was reserved for men. Female saints—no matter how great their learning, wisdom, service, or piety—had to have been virgins or martyrs or both.

revered by some, they were simply eclipsed and forgotten. In the eyes of many, every woman was an Eve, a temptress, best kept behind doors, silent and submissive.

The fact is that the early Christian church was closer to a crowd than a choir. There was not as yet any theological equivalent of "perfect pitch," much less a hymnal. Consensus was simply not a foreseeable nor even a sought-after option. That said, as good Romans the early Christians knew the worth of a straight road and were resolved to do their best to build one as they hammered out their core doctrines. Orthodoxy was an obsession with them, and so they were prepared to level or remove every obstacle in its path. Another Roman imperial value not left behind was the commitment to a clear and strict hierarchy of power and authority, and so a clerical, theological elite emerged, an outspoken self-elected quorum that silenced the radical fringe and sidelined the silent majority. The resulting paradox is that while Christians in the Roman Empire at the close of the second century may have numbered as many as five million, relatively few of their voices or views have survived. Instead, for better or for worse, we must mostly rely on a vocal minority of history's choosing to inform us of the early Christian's ideas and practices regarding the morality or immorality of sexuality and warfare.

It might be argued that for the earliest Christians the question whether having sex and making war could be moral acts was preempted by the question whether these activities were even necessary. True enough, without marriage Rome's population would plummet, and without the military the empire's borders would collapse. But both of these calamities would take time, and time was precisely what, in the starry eyes of many first- and second-century Christian believers, neither Rome nor the world had. Truly one of the banner headlines of the gospels was the announcement that "the kingdom of heaven has come near" (Matt 10:7) and that it is not of this world. Many believed and took to heart what Jesus had said of "those who belong to this age," how "they marry and are given in marriage; but those who are considered worthy of a place in that age and in the resurrection from the dead neither marry nor are given in marriage" (Luke 20:34–35). With the drawing near of the divine bridegroom and the dawn of his eternal reign so close at hand, it seemed no time to snuff out the lights and take to the private intimacy of one's bed; rather it was time to light a lamp and keep constant vigil, for "truly I tell you, you will not have gone through all the towns of Israel before the Son of Man comes" (Matt 10:23). There is no way to know just how many of Christianity's first and most fervent or fearful converts embraced the eschatological vision of an imminent end of days. While we know that some did, we would not be far off the mark in assuming that others continued to plow their fields, patch their roofs, sleep with their mates, and raise their children to take up where they would leave off.

The "present age" or *saeculum* in which the earliest missionaries of Christ awakened to their calling was, of course, the age of imperial Rome, whose cities, roads, prosperity, linguistic homogeneity, and internal security provided fortuitous—some would say providential—soil for the germination and growth of the nascent Christian church. The first Christians and their *ecclesiae* or gatherings were, in large part, urban—centered in one or other of the great Roman cities of the Eastern Mediterranean and Near East, cities such as Ephesus, Antioch, Thessalonica, Corinth, Alexandria, and Rome. For these first Christians, service in the Roman legions was not a probable option and therefore not a pressing issue. Marriage, on the other hand, was more obligatory than optional. With an average life expectancy of less than twenty-five years and with only 4 percent of the male population living past fifty years of age, heirs were, like water, a matter of household survival.[2] For any extended family or household to preserve its identity, influence, lands, and wealth, it required legitimate progeny and especially sons; and, beyond the household, on the imperial scale, fruitful sex was a patriotic necessity. In simple numbers, a Roman woman reaching the age of fifteen would have to bear in her lifetime a mean of roughly five children, if the society were to hope to maintain its current population. Well aware of the crisis implied in these numbers and leaving no doubt regarding the link between sex and citizenship, Augustus twice enacted legislation (the *lex Julia* in 18 BCE and the *lex Papia Poppaea* in 9 CE) that "enforced various civil disabilities on those not marrying and not having children."[3]

It tended to be at the extreme edges of the faith and of the empire, then, that lifelong celibacy was openly embraced and touted by arresting and often eloquent world-renouncing zealots, who regarded procreation as, among other things, collaboration with the *saeculum*, the secular reign of death whose certain and imminent demise had already been declared by Jesus of Nazareth. "To break the spell of the bed was to break the spell of

---

2. See Burn, "*Hic Breve Vivitur*," for a discussion of this topic.

3. Frier, "Roman Life Expectancy," 249.

the world."[4] While these radical celibates, such as Tatian and his Encratite followers, remained on the fringe of Christian practice, their dark and dismissive views of sexuality were moving into the mainstream. Intercourse and procreation, once simple and not unwelcome facts of life, were now seen as profoundly problematic and suspect. On the face of it, the intimacies of sex would appear to offer some respite from the weariness of life's everyday labors, while the resulting offspring stand as an investment in life and a consolation in the face of personal mortality. Instead, Christians came to see their mortal bodies as seedbeds of corruption, binding them to death and to the inherent sinfulness that is death's cause and consort. In fact, according to the third-century Syriac manuscript, the *Didascalia Apostolorum* or "Teachings of the Apostles," sexual intercourse, menstruation, and nocturnal emissions were all seen as pollutants and so as grounds for exclusion from the Eucharist and all things holy.[5] Similarly, the second canon of Archbishop and Saint Dionysius of Alexandria stated that "menstruous women ought not to come to the Holy Table, or touch the Holy of Holies, nor to churches, but pray elsewhere."[6] Christian life, ignited like a new flame in baptism, was meant to be free from bondage to sin and death, and this came to mean a life of the spirit free from the urges, necessities, delights, and delusions of carnal existence. Not surprisingly, sex epitomized "the flesh" and its fatal allurements. Flesh, even in the flowering of sexual delight and fecundity, had about it now the stench of death. As Peter Brown makes brilliantly clear,

> The new way of thinking that emerged in Christian circles in the course of the second century shifted the center of gravity of thought on the nature of human frailty from death to sexuality. For sexual desire was no longer presented as a benign remedy for death. Some Christian thinkers presented it as the first cause of death. Others, less drastic, saw it as the first, most blatant manifestation of Adam and Eve's loss of the immortality conferred on them by possession of God's Spirit. For all, sexuality edged itself into the center of attention, as a privileged symptom of humanity's fall into bondage. Consequently, the renunciation of sexual intercourse came to be linked on a deep symbolic level with the

4. Brown, *Body and Society*, 98.

5. See *Didascalia Apostolorum* 26.6.21.

6. Dionysius of Alexandria, Canon 2, in response to letter from Basilides the bishop; cited by O'Grady, "Sematics of Taboo," 12. This prohibition is all the more incongruous and shocking when placed beside the story of the "unclean" woman in Mark 5:25–34.

reestablishment of a lost human freedom, with a regaining of the Spirit of God, and, so, with man's ability to undo the power of death.[7]

It would be no slight task to trace a straight intelligible path from the Jesus of the gospels to the ferocious Christian renunciates of the second century and beyond. Jesus appeared for the most part at home in his body, while many early Christians were hardly at peace in theirs. Their faith-driven dis-ease in their own flesh, and their conviction that to embrace the incarnate God meant to become somehow disincarnate themselves, defy any simple argument or logic. What these clearly reflect, however, is the rich and riotous philosophical and religious gene pool from which Christianity initially surfaced. Jewish Essenes, Valentinian Gnostics, Roman Stoics, Oriental Manichaeans, Indian Buddhists, Greek Neoplatonists, to mention a few, all form a part of the early Christian genome. In these circles let it be said that the body, much less its most notorious organs, had few firm friends or proponents. The best we can do here, and what will suffice for our purposes, is to continue to describe the broadest conflicts waged and conclusions reached in the first centuries of Christianity regarding sex and marriage, for this will shed appreciable and unexpected light on the early church's proclamations and policies regarding the waging of war.

No matter how vocal were the proponents of lifelong abstinence, needless to say sex retained a solid majority of more or less silent supporters, even among the clergy. After all, as Paul and other half-hearted defenders of marriage pointed out, married sex was preferable to uncontrolled fornication. "For it is better to marry," conceded Paul to the Christian community at Corinth, "than to be aflame with passion" (1 Cor 7:9). That said, the sexless life came to be the Christian ideal, towards which even "half-Christians" or married couples might and should, by degree, aspire. It need not be all or nothing. Compromise was possible, and compromise took multiple forms. One was to confine sex and procreation to youth and the early years of marriage, when desire is greatest and fertility most predictable. This route resembled and may even have been influenced by the *ashrama dharma* of Hinduism, according to which the righteous man progresses from householder to forest dweller to renunciate, thus assuring not only the continuity of family and society but also his own movement towards spiritual perfection and liberation. In the meantime, sex was to be for the purpose of propagation, not pleasure. This called for rare discipline

7. Brown, *Body and Society,* 86.

and careful planning. At the very least it meant that the intention to propagate be foremost in the minds of both partners in sex, and their attraction to one another altogether secondary.[8] Ajax of Gaza surely stood as both a prodigy and a poster child of near perfectly chaste marriage; for "although he had an exceptionally beautiful wife, he slept with her on only three occasions, producing three boys, two of whom became monks, leaving the third to carry on the family name!"[9] Even beyond controlling the frequency of intercourse and making propagation its prevailing intent, some aspired even further to the still more ascetically ambitious state of *apatheia*, the absence of appetite, sex without desire (*non concupsicere*), an achievement that Clement of Alexandria, its proponent, admitted was impossible without the grace of God.[10]

Meanwhile, in the late third century, a new flame of fervor was struck and burned bright on the Christian spiritual landscape—the monastic movement. Once again radical, world-renouncing Christianity took root in the desert, in the wilderness rather than in the cities. The lives and legends of Antony, Pachomius, and Basil of Caesarea and all those who followed them into remote yet luminous austerity provided ordinary lay Christians with a shining ideal to which they would never live up but to which they would always look up. These were their barely incarnate angels, their guardian angels, to whom they turned for intercession and counsel. It may be said that the Christian church, from its beginnings, focused itself on two questions: "Who was the Christ?" and "Who is the Christian?" The first was a theological concern, to be debated and decided in the early ecumenical councils. The second was a matter of practice and had more to do with how to live and die than with what to think. In some ways this had been clear from the start. Christians were to imitate Christ, to live as he had lived and to die as he had died, so that they might hope to rise as he had risen. Consequently, martyrs provided the paradigm. The word *martus* means "witness," and Christian martyrs bore the ultimate witness to Christ, in their agonies and in their blood, shed as his blood had been shed for the remission of sins and the salvation of humankind.

8. We may safely assume that this was not the sort of sex that Augustine engaged in with his lover of thirteen years, since in all that time together they produced but one child. Perhaps it was his own sexual experience that led Augustine to break ranks with so many more rigorous and reprimanding clerics and submit the opinion that sex for pleasure, within marriage, is a "pardonable" fault.

9. Brown, *Body and Society*, 325.

10. Clement, *Stromateis*, 3.7.57.

Not all Christians, however, were willing to be martyrs, and not all those who were willing received the opportunity. Despite their front-page notoriety, deadly persecutions were few, fierce, and far between. Martyrdom—the self-sacrificial imitation of and witnessing to Christ—had to adopt other forms. Tertullian—often labeled "the Father of Latin Christianity"—saw in chastity, the renunciation of the flesh, an available alternative form of authentic martyrdom or life-denying witness. This very witness came to full fruition in the lives of the desert monks, male and female, who embraced what came to been seen as "white" or bloodless martyrdom, a laying down of their lives that stopped short of literal suicide. They only imitated death and, in doing so, sought to imitate Christ. They ate and slept, clothed themselves and took shelter, but only to the extent required to sustain life, a life of constant, vigilant prayer. In the imaginations of the ordinary faithful, however, it was their chastity, their renunciation of sexual desire and delight, that was their brightest flame, burning away sin and corruption and casting a beam by which they measured their own compromised lives.

Renouncing sex and marriage, however, was not on the table (much less in the bed) for the majority of Christians. Rome was an empire of households, and the Christian church too, despite all its monks and hermits, was essentially comprised of families that were the indispensable seedbeds of the future. Without them there could be no future at all, and the truth was that, as the centuries progressed, the church put behind it the apocalyptic expectations of its infancy and became ever more deeply invested in the New Age, the Christian Age. In this new imperium, however, the laity or "the worldly" (*kosmikoi*), tainted with sex and secularity, were disqualified for leadership so long as they slept in marriage beds. This meant, as noted earlier, that those who had married in their youth might later vow themselves to chastity, having already produced and reared their children; and indeed a number of the most influential early saints and church leaders took this very path, leading to what Peter Brown referred to as "a Spirit-filled gerontocracy"[11] in the early church. By the time of Augustine and Ambrose, Jerome and Eusebius, the Christian church had long affirmed yet only imperfectly implemented its two-caste system: a majority of lay men and women living in "the world" and largely consumed with its demands and responsibilities; and a spiritually "ruling" minority of "otherworldly" celibate clergy, monks, and nuns living apart, in cloisters of one sort or

11. Brown, *Body and Society,* 79.

another, officially above and exempt from the necessities of secular existence—necessities that include, of course, sex and military service, without which the next generation would neither exist nor survive. Lest we imagine that this system came from the minds of mere men, Eusebius, bishop of Caesarea in the early fourth century, wished to make it quite clear that the separation of the flock into shepherds and sheep was ordained by the Son of God himself:

> Two ways of life were thus given by the law of Christ to His Church. The one is above nature, and beyond common human living; it admits not marriage, child-bearing, property nor the possession of wealth, but wholly and permanently separate from the common customary life of mankind, it devotes itself to the service of God alone in its wealth of heavenly love! And they who enter on this course, appear to die to the life of mortals, to bear with them nothing earthly but their body, and in mind and spirit to have passed to heaven . . . performing the duty of a priesthood to Almighty God for the whole race. . . . Such then is the perfect form of the Christian life. And the other more humble, more human, permits men to join in pure nuptials and to produce children, to undertake government, to give orders to soldiers fighting for right; it allows them to have minds for farming, for trade, and the other more secular interests as well as for religion. . . . And a kind of secondary grade of piety is attributed to them, giving just such help as such lives require.[12]

While it remained the case for centuries that many clergy, especially those in smaller towns and villages, slept with their wives, celebrated Mass, and administered the sacraments without contradiction, such figures were marginal and belonged to the past. The future of the church belonged to the celibate elite, who were declared to be the foundation of the church.

Before we turn to the issue of military service, we would do well to sum up the conclusions reached by the early Christian church regarding the moral legitimacy of sex and marriage. The first point to be made is that for the most part the church recognized and acknowledged that "someone has to do it." In other words, sex is necessary. On the other hand it is corrupting and discrediting, that is, it is always more or less sinful: more sinful when passionate and motivated by desire, less sinful when dispassionate and controlled by the intention to procreate. This being the case, sex and procreation were assigned to a Christian subclass, who despite their vastly

12. Eusebius of Caesarea, *Demonstration*, 1:8.

superior numbers are subject in all things spiritual to a minority of celibates who have foresworn the polluting, carnal taint and tug of sex.

Having witnessed the ancient entanglement of sex and violence in the ancient imagination, it should come as no surprise to find that the early Christian church's evolving policies and practices regarding military service rather precisely parallel its policies and practices regarding marriage. That is to say that military service, though incompatible with the Christian life, is at the same time a worldly necessity. Once again, "someone has to do it," which doesn't make it right, only unavoidable. Killing, the consummate act of the military (like sex, the consummate rite of marriage), is always polluting and more or less sinful: more sinful when passionate and driven by rage or revenge, less sinful when controlled by the intention to protect the empire and punish its enemies. Those who undertake this bloody responsibility, however, like those tainted with sex, are given only limited access to the sacred and no access at all to Holy Orders. The clergy are to be without taint, without sin, without pollution, which means that they are to be both celibate and nonviolent; for only the virgin and the pacifist bear true and perfect witness to Christ. In saying this now, however, we are ahead of ourselves in our discussion. We need, instead, to trace the development of the church's views on war and military service through the first centuries of the Common Era.

It is clear from the outset that the question of Christian military service—whether Christian faith and military service are mutually compatible—is a good deal more charged and complex than the question of Christian sexuality and marriage. Of the three sins deemed "irremissable" by Tertullian and the early Fathers—idolatry, adultery, and homicide—two were occupational requirements for Roman legionnaires. Service in the legions was inescapably idolatrous, as the Roman army had its own religion, encompassing nearly every aspect of a soldier's life—its own rituals, deities, cult objects, religious festivals, and sacred oaths. The core military oath, taken by every soldier upon enlistment and twice annually from then on, was called the *sacramentum*, the same term used by the early Christian church for baptism and the Eucharist. This oath was made to the emperor, the *pontifex maximus* or high priest of the Roman state religion, and represented in the eyes of many early Christians a pact with the devil.[13] Likewise, while some soldiers had only administrative duties, most were in the business of combat and killing, and there was no space in the early church

13. See Tertullian, *On Idolatry*, 19.315.

between this killing and homicide. In fact, holding any reasonably high public office in the empire often involved the administration of justice and thus of capital punishment, which also qualified as homicide in the eyes of most Christians. The category of legal murder made sense to the state but not to the early church. Consequently, though our focus here is on military service, much of what we will discuss applied as well to government service more generally understood.

The earliest Christian church was unevenly divided in its opinion of and loyalty to the Roman Empire. Some identified Rome with "Babylon the great, mother of whores and of earth's abominations" (Rev 17:5) and the Antichrist of the book of Revelation, but a more accommodating and even appreciative view of the empire prevailed among Christians, especially when the emperor was not unleashing a persecution against them. After all, Rome, in providing civil order and protection, made the world safe for Christianity, allowing it to grow and flourish. In his Epistle to the Romans, Paul made a point that would be made many times again through the centuries, when he urged every Christian to "be subject to the governing authorities" on the grounds that "there is no authority except from God, and those authorities that exist have been instituted by God. Therefore whoever resists authority resists what God has appointed. . . . For rulers are not a terror to good conduct, but to bad" (Rom 13:1–3). This expressive vote of confidence in the state only widened as the hope for an imminent end-of-days waned and gave way, instead, to a deep fear of the apocalypse and of the unthinkable catastrophe it would entail. The church that had once prayed for the timely return of Christ in the second coming now commonly found itself wishing and even praying for a delay.[14] Christians, it seems, were in no hurry for the present age to come to an end, nor for the Pax Romana to come crashing down.

Even a vociferous and unyielding opponent of Christian military service such as Tertullian could find it in himself to pray not only for the health and longevity of the emperor but also for the success of the empire in its endeavors, including its military campaigns. "Without ceasing," he writes in his *Apology* (ca. 197), addressed to Emperor Septimius Severus,

> for all our emperors we offer prayer. We pray for life prolonged;
> for security to the empire; for protection to the imperial house; for

14. See Tertullian, *Apology* 39.2.

brave armies, a faithful senate, a virtuous people, the world at rest, whatever, as man or Caesar, an emperor would wish.[15]

The broader point that Tertullian was making in his *Apology* was that Christians made good Roman citizens and were loyal to the state. At the same time, Christians kept their distance from Roman temples and found it difficult to go to war, given their belief that it was more permissible for them to be killed than to kill. While Tertullian acknowledged that Christians were currently serving in the military, he was more than uneasy about this fact. While some had made a distinction between soldiers who converted to Christianity and Christians who signed up for the military, this was a distinction lost on Tertullian. He found it impossible to reconcile Christianity with service as a soldier, a governor, or a magistrate, for these offices placed the soul of the Christian in grave peril, requiring as they did both lethal and idolatrous behavior. The only minor and reluctant concession uttered by Tertullian was his admission that Christians already in the army, who would face desertion charges should they simply walk away, might remain there so as long as they take no part in a single act of violence or idolatry.

The challenges posed by imperial service were nothing new in the late second and early third centuries, and by then an unknown number of Christians had doubtless made their own private peace with a career in the legions or in the Roman civil service. The truth is that this number was growing. Despite that fact, Tertullian appears to have been the first to bring this issue to front stage in the early Christian forum and to call the question, as it were, on whether Christians could ever legitimately shed the blood of others. For him, the answer was easy. With clear reference to the gospel episode relating how Jesus, on the night of his arrest, had reproved and disarmed Peter after he had cut off the right ear of the high priest, Tertullian asked, "How will a Christian go to war or for that matter how will he serve even in peace, without a sword that the Lord has taken away? . . . In disarming Peter, the Lord disarmed every future soldier. No uniform is lawful among us, if it stands for sinful action."[16]

Tertullian's indictment of Christian military and civil service was sharp and unyielding. The inescapable reality for Christians was that they cannot serve two masters and that through baptism they are enlisted in the forces of light, not those of darkness. The notion that killing for the

15. Tertullian, *Apology*, 30.4.

16. Tertullian, *On Idolatry*, 19.318, 321. Adapted from the 1885 translation by S. Thelwall.

state constituted a special category of legitimate or ethical bloodshed was in his judgment sheer delusion and avoidance, as was any plea made on the grounds of necessity. "A state of faith admits no plea of necessity," wrote Tertullian in *De Corona* (*The Chaplet*). "They [Christians] are under no necessity to sin, whose one necessity is that they do not sin."[17] Christian soldiers and imperial officials are without excuse for the positions they hold, the authorities they answer to, and the functions they perform. It is one thing to pray for the emperor and his men in arms or in the purple, and quite another to serve in their ranks.

Tertullian was hardly alone in his opposition to Christian service in an imperial system that enforced its laws, expanded and maintained its borders, and punished its criminals and enemies with lethal force. The deep and widely held Christian aversion to bloodshed and thus to such service soon found canonical expression in a contemporary document known as the *Apostolic Tradition*. This text, long attributed to Hippolytus of Rome,[18] belongs to the genre of early church writings known as "Ancient Church Orders," which proposed to address with apostolic authority a range of matters dealing with liturgy, morals, and ecclesiastical discipline. Presumably, its declarations on military service and other related matters carried some weight in the church at a time when the number of Christians in military service was increasing. This latter fact was an aberration that, according to this document, was not to be tolerated:

> A soldier of the civil authority must be taught not to kill men and to refuse to do so if he is commanded, and to refuse to take an oath; if he is unwilling to comply, he must be rejected [by the Christian church]. A military commander or civic magistrate that wears the purple must resign or be rejected [by the church]. If a catechumen or a believer seeks to become a soldier, they must be rejected, for they have despised God.[19]

Cyprian, Tertullian's successor in Carthage, though less decisive or outspoken on the issue of military service, nevertheless contributed this cutting commentary on the often glossed over criminality of state-sanctioned killing:

17. Tertullian, *The Chaplet*, 11.421.

18. The authorship but not the antiquity of this document has been strongly contested in recent years.

19. Hippolytus, *Apostolic Tradition*, II.16.17–19.

The whole world is wet with mutual blood; and murder, which in the case of an individual is admitted to be a crime, is called a virtue when it is committed wholesale. Impunity is claimed for the wicked deeds, not on the plea that they are guiltless, but because the cruelty is perpetrated on a grand scale.[20]

In another of his writings, Cyprian adds that manslaughter is a mortal crime, an act that kills the soul of the killer, and so the hands of those who have received the Eucharist must never allow themselves to be stained with the blood of others.[21]

We will conclude this discussion of the predominantly though not unanimously pacifist[22] views and voices of the early Christian church with Origen Adamantius of Alexandria, widely acknowledged to be the most deeply learned and dazzling Christian scholar of the first three centuries. A story told by Eusebius of Caesarea relates how Origen might easily have perished as a teenager at the time of the Emperor Septimius Severus, when his father Leonides was martyred for his faith and when Origen would willingly have followed his father to an untimely death had his mother not hidden his clothes. Denied martyrdom, he is said to have taken quite literally the challenge posed in the Gospel of Matthew and made himself a eunuch for "the sake of the kingdom of heaven" (19:12), thus embracing a life of surgically irreversible celibacy. Not surprisingly, his views on killing were no less uncompromising and adamant than his views on sex.

It was Origen who took it on himself to pen a belated response to Celsus, a Platonist critic who, under the title "The True Word" (*alethes logos*), had published an extensive frontal attack on Christianity that, amidst a wide range of accusations, had questioned the loyalty and patriotism of Christians. Though composed at least a half-century earlier when Origen was a mere child, Celsus' tract had lost none of its relevance or sting; so Origen took it on in his own countertreatise entitled *Contra Celsum*, which might colloquially be translated "Back at Celsus." Among the charges filed by Celsus was that Christians had for centuries enjoyed and prospered

---

20. Cyprian of Carthage, *Epistles*, 1.6.

21. See Cyprian of Carthage, *Treatises*, 9.14.

22. A notable exception to the pacifist Christian chorus of the first three centuries was Clement of Alexandria, a towering church leader in the late second and early third centuries. Both on the question of Christian marriage and on that of Christian military service, Clement sought to chart a moderate course. While upholding the spiritual primacy of chastity and peace, he held back from altogether denouncing either marriage or military service.

within the safe haven made possible by the empire and its legions but had refused to bear their fair share of the burden of maintaining the empire's security and good order. Peace, in other words, comes at a price, and Christians had shown themselves unwilling to pay that price, most pointedly by refusing to serve in the empire's army.

The truth is that Celsus was not well informed regarding the fact that even as he wrote there were indeed Christians serving in the military and that their number was growing. Origen knew this and knew as well that Christian enlistment in the military as well as military converts to Christianity had increased at an even greater rate in the ensuing years since Celsus had filed his complaint. But this was not something that Origen approved of and it would not form the basis of his response. Instead, he endeavored to make the case that Christians provided the empire and its legions with an even greater service than that of bearing arms. What the church offers the empire is the incomparably greater boon of divine assistance delivered through the intercessory power of its prayers. "To be sure," argues Origen,

> the holier a man is, the more effective help does he render to emperors, even more than is given by soldiers, who go forth to fight and kill as many of the enemy as they can. And to those enemies of our faith who require us to bear arms for the common good, and to kill men, we can reply: Do not those who are priests at certain shrines, and those who attend on certain gods, as you account them, keep their hands free from blood, that they may with hands unstained and free from human blood offer the appointed sacrifices to your gods; and even when war is upon you, you never enlist the priests in the army. If that, then, is a laudable custom, how much more so, that while others are engaged in battle, these too should engage as the priests and ministers of God, keeping their hands pure, and wrestling in prayers to God on behalf of those who are fighting in a righteous cause, and for the emperor who reigns righteously, that whatever is opposed to those who act righteously may be destroyed![23]

The case made by Origen for Christian pacifism was both canny and prophetic. In *Contra Celsum*, Origen acknowledged the legitimacy of the emperor's concerns for the security and well-being of his people as well as the legitimacy of his exercising lethal force to accomplish those ends. In other words, Origen recognized that there was a proper time and place for

23. Origen, *Against Celsus*, 8.73. Adapted from the 1885 translation by Frederick Crombie.

war and killing, a time when lethal force was necessary and just, in human secular terms. In the same breath, however, he claimed Christian exemption from any direct participation in such acts, on the same grounds as the priests of Roman civil religion enjoyed a similar exemption. In asserting this equivalency, Origen is clearly claiming that all Christians share in the priesthood of Christ and are a holy people, nonviolent to their core; for Jesus "nowhere teaches that it is right for his own disciples to offer violence to anyone, however wicked. For he did not deem it in keeping with such laws as his, which were derived from a divine source, to allow the killing of any individual whatever."[24] Rules are rules, and divine law preempts civil law. Of all people, the Romans, who defend the purity of their own priests and know why they do this, ought to grasp why they need respect the priestly purity of all Christians and not expect them to stain their hands and their souls with bloodshed. Origen must have realized that the case he was making here was more than the average Roman, much less the emperor, could swallow. In fact, it was also more than the church—drawing an ever-broader line between clergy and laity—was prepared to embrace.

In his counterattack on Celsus, Origen had made a novel point. He highlighted a significant difference between the "necessity" of marriage and the "necessity" of military service. The church, without blessing sexuality, had made room for marriage by assigning it to the laity, the worldly underclass of half-Christians who accepted their marginality in return for the pleasures of intimacy and the comforts of family. This deal was necessary if the church was to flourish through the centuries, because it could not and would not rely, for its survival and growth, on the conversion of other people's offspring. The pagan Romans were in no position, much less were they inclined, to be surrogate parents for a celibate Christian church. Christians were going to have to have their own sex and their own babies, but not, as we have seen, all Christians.

It was a different matter, in Origen's view, when it came to waging war. Here, he argued, Christians can and must expect pagan Romans to do their fighting for them. Impossible as it was to imagine a universally celibate church, Origen considered it not at all impossible, but in fact incumbent on all believers, to envision and become a universally pacifist church. After all, as not only he saw it, the Christian church is a pilgrim church, a community in this world but not of this world, a church with staff in hand on its way to the City of God. In the meantime—however long that may prove to be—the

24. Ibid., 3.7.

church can and should go forth and multiply but need not and should not erect its own earthly empire in order to defend itself against the forces of evil. It has both the legions of Rome and the legions of God's angels to do that for it.

Looking back over the first three centuries of Christianity, then, when the church first confronted on its own terms the most urgent and universal desires and fears of its members and thus the unavoidable and entwined issues of sexuality and violence, we have seen that the case for Christian pacifism was more easily made and widely embraced than the case for celibacy. Unlike the case against marriage and for virginity, the argument for Christian pacifism found ample, direct support in the life and words of Jesus, as found in the four gospels. That Jesus of Nazareth was a nonviolent man of peace who went to his own violent death, not with arms swinging but with arms willingly outstretched, is a fact lost on no one who reads the New Testament with an open mind. He blessed "the peacemakers" (Matt 5:9) not the warriors, and opposed the exercise of violence, even in self-defense or revenge, instructing his disciples in no uncertain terms: "Do not resist the evil-doer. But if anyone strikes you on the right cheek, turn the other also. . . . Love your enemies and pray for those who persecute you" (Matt 5:39, 44; cf. Luke 6:27–36). Clearly, this was a lesson that Jesus not only spoke but also lived. As evidence of this we have already noted how it was that Jesus disavowed Peter's use of violent force in the garden at the time of his arrest, taking away his sword and replacing at once the ear that Peter had sliced off. That said, there were those who—seeking to condone or even call for the righteous exercise of Christian violence—combed the Scriptures, Jewish and Christian, for inspired support and claimed to have found enough to make their case; but it was a case that failed to convince the majority of outspoken Christians, particularly in the Hellenistic East, until the unthinkable occurred in the Christian conversion of the Emperor Constantine and the evil empire became, overnight as it were, holy.

5

Christian Rome

Warriors and Saints

I N THE EARLY CHURCH, Christianity was all about conversion. Jesus, it might be said, "converted" his first disciples, and they in turn were sent out to convert the nations of the earth. Of all the conversions of the first century the most notorious and consequential was surely that of Saul, unseated from his horse on the road to Damascus by a blinding beam of light and stunned to silence by the voice of the same Jesus whose followers he was so busy persecuting (Acts 9:3–9). It is safe to say of this moment that Saul never saw it coming and had no idea where it would lead. Where it led, of course, was Christianity, a religion whose members, by the fourth century, numbered in the millions.

For all their numbers, however, Christians were hardly safe and sound within their churches and homes. The early fourth century was again a time of bitter persecution, this time the Great Persecution of Diocletian, whose scale and ferocity were both unprecedented and later exaggerated by Christian authors. Hyperbole aside, the series of persecutory edicts issued by Diocletian and the other members of his imperial Tetrarchy stripped Christians of their legal rights, burned their assemblies and holy books, confiscated their property, and required them to sacrifice to the pagan gods. For a number of reasons, ranging from uneven enforcement to opportune compliance to simply lying low, the vast majority of Christians survived this period of terror, though not without fresh divisions among them.

Lactantius, among the most learned and influential Christian authors of his generation, saw in the Great Persecution the coming of the Apocalypse. What he and his contemporaries did not see coming was the conversion of Constantine and the consequent birth of Christendom.

The conversion experience of Flavius Valerius Aurelius Constantinus Augustus was no more subtle than that of Saint Paul, at least in the accounts that have come down to us from Lactantius and Eusebius, the latter account dictated to Eusebius years later under oath by the emperor himself. Constantine was at the time an Augustus at war, on the brink of a decisive battle, stopped in his tracks by a luminous cross appearing overhead in the noonday sky and bearing the inscription "in this sign you will conquer." Then, as if this were not enough to move him, that same night he was visited by a second vision in which Jesus commanded him to have his men paint the *labarum* or Chi-Rho—the first two Greek letters in the name "Christ"—on their shields and so to advance against the enemy with the sign of Christ as their military standard. The next day, on October 28, 312, in the Battle of the Milvian Bridge, Constantine, with a force half the size of his opponent's, defeated his rival Maxentius and, like Moses, Joshua, and David before him, witnessed the awful force of the Lord of Hosts, "who trains my hands for war, and my fingers for battle" (Ps 144:1).

This victory, won under the battle standard of Christ, set Constantine on a sure path to sole imperial power and at the same time assured Christianity not only a place of security but also a position of privilege within the empire. While it is not possible to mark the precise moment when Constantine "became Christian"—his baptism seemingly delayed until shortly before his death—the bond between him and the church was clear and grew ever more manifest in the years following his visions and victory at the Milvian Bridge. Beginning with the Edict of Milan in 313, in which he and his eastern counterpart Licinius rescinded all persecutory and prejudicial legislation against Christians and restored their confiscated property and wealth, Constantine continued to reveal and to write into law his special favor for the Christian religion and its adherents. Even further, he used his authority and clout to help cauterize the internal wounds within the church that were in part the legacy of the long persecution that he had at one time condoned. When, in 324, Constantine finally ruled absolute over a united empire, and the church stood more intact than it had been within anyone's memory, Christians might easily have imagined that the kingdom of God was at hand. Clearly they saw the hand of their Savior in Constantine's rise to power and in his conversion. Bishop Eusebius of Caesarea, the euphoric personal biographer of Constantine, described him as "the Servant of God and the Conqueror of Nations,"[1] and saw the emperor as indeed God's "friend, graced by his heavenly favor with victory over all his foes."[2] True enough, from its infancy the Christian church had more or less consistently regarded the Roman emperor as an unwitting providential agent of their God, providing the soil and the infrastructure, as it were, for the spread of the faith and the development of its own institutions. But Constantine was different, radically so; for he was in fact the knowing ally, even the faithful friend, of the Christian God. Christians now saw the empire as their very own, as the willing and able consort of the Holy Church.

Drawing in this account, now, to a tighter focus on the particular concerns of this book, it is crucial to note that Constantine was no man of peace. He had risen through the ranks of the military and, upon the death of his father, Flavius Constantius, had been acclaimed Augustus by his own legions. From there he had battled his way to the top, eliminating his competition by the sword. Furthermore, the particular Christ who came to him and won him to his side, like the God of the Jewish Scriptures, was no more a pacifist than he was. Rather, he enlisted Constantine and his army and led them, with his holy standard, into battle and to victory. There is perhaps no more graphic or poignant illustration of the full legitimation of state violence in the Christian empire of Constantine than the fact that when Constantine's mother, Saint Helena, brought back from the Holy Land a cache of most sacred relics, including several nails believed to have been the very ones used to affix Jesus to his cross, he had these melted down and incorporated into his battle helmet and into the bridle-bits for his war horse.[3]

The decidedly marshal proclivities and prowess of Constantine appear to have come as no disappointment, much less a scandal, to the Christian church in the fourth century. After all, these were exceedingly violent and dangerous times, and Constantine was well suited to them. The fate of the empire and that of the church were now entwined, and—it was feared—both lay in peril. In retrospect, we know that such fears were well grounded. In less than a century, the Eternal City of Rome would fall to the Visigoths, and in less than two centuries the Roman state and army would cease to

1. Eusebius, *Life of Constantine*, I.6.
2. Eusebius, *Oration*, II.3.
3. Socrates Scholasticus, *Ecclesiastical History*, I.17

exist. To call the conversion of Constantine a turning point in the Christian church's position on war and military service barely states the fact. Nearly overnight, the case for pacifism was forgotten. Was it a matter of mortal fear, imperial fervor, or even a new and blatant Christian jingoism? It may even be that the roots of Christian nonviolence had never run all that deep in the first place. However we might explain or fail to explain it, the mind and heart of the church on the exercise of violence and the matter of killing changed with surprising suddenness, a change that can be traced quite clearly in the writings of Lactantius, who at one point stated quite unequivocally that

> when God forbids us to kill, He not only prohibits us from open violence, which is not even allowed by the public laws, but He warns us against the commission of those things which are es-teemed lawful among men. Thus it will be neither lawful for a just man to engage in warfare, since his warfare is justice itself, nor to accuse any one of a capital charge, because it makes no difference whether you put a man to death by word, or rather by the sword, since it is the act of putting to death itself which is prohibited. Therefore, with regard to this precept of God, there ought to be no exception at all; but that it is always unlawful to put to death a man, whom God willed to be a sacred animal.[4]

Yet, at another and later point, the same man found it within himself to write with equal conviction regarding "the passions"—anger, love of gain, and sexual desire—that they ought not to be taken away nor lessened:

> For they are not evil of themselves, since God has reasonably implanted them in us; but inasmuch as they are plainly good by nature,—for they are given us for the protection of life,—they be-come evil by their evil use. And as bravery, if you fight in defense of your country, is a good, if against your country, is an evil, so the passions, if you employ them to good purposes, will be virtues, if to evil uses, they will be called vices.[5]

Lactantius, in a former life, as it were, had lived and written in fear for his life during the Great Persecution. Then, only a handful of years later, he was addressing his work to the emperor himself and eventually won an imperial appointment as court tutor to Constantine's son. Change—at this pace and extreme—is indeed mind-bending. And so it was for the church

4. Lactantius. *Divine Institutes*, VI.20.15–17.
5. Lactantius, *Epitome*, LXI.3–4.

whose most eminent scholars and spokesmen of the fourth century bent their minds anew around the question of war and killing and came up with moral and theological justifications for both. At the same time, military service—so far from being suspect, if not flat-out forbidden, for Christians—was becoming a matter of Christian duty. In fact, only a century after the conversion of Constantine, military service, by imperial decree, was the exclusive prerogative of Christians. No non-Christians need apply.

It was not Christian bishops and theologians, like Ambrose and Augustine, who first invented or invoked the concept of just war, that is, war waged for a legitimate reason and in a legitimate manner. Even a cursory survey of ancient literature, law, and history will turn up innumerable examples of warriors and statesmen attempting to justify their wars, either in prospect or in retrospect. War is one of those things that doesn't go without saying or pass without inspection. But for Christians, the problem was different and deeper than for most others who took pause before taking life. Christians were sworn by their baptismal oath to follow in the footsteps of a man whose life and message came down to one word: love. Confronted with violence, they were to turn the other cheek. They were to love their enemies and not to resist evil, any more than he had when seized and nailed to a cross. This was the new commandment, the new law that eclipsed all others. And this was the obstacle that theologians faced when attempting to construct a Christian case for killing, state killing, whether in war or in a court of law. Until the fourth century a Christian empire was an oxymoron. Now it was a challenge. However unthinkable it was to imagine a Christian army, it was even more of a stretch to entertain the idea of a nonviolent empire.

It was Ambrose of Milan and his protégé Augustine of Hippo who constructed the bridge—a characteristically durable Roman bridge—from the pacifism of the New Testament to the militarism of post-Constantinian Christianity. Both were ambitious men of the world, bent on political advancement in an imperial bureaucracy whose responsibilities and demands they accepted. They took for granted the partnership of church and state forged by Constantine, who had died before either of them was born. They were, at the same time, intellectual giants and fervent Christians who at a critical point in their respective careers changed course and rose to authority within the church rather than in the state, although at the time these represented two sides of the same street. Closer to our focal concerns here is the fact that in envisioning just war Augustine stood on Ambrose's shoulders, at once relying on and surpassing his mentor. Both believed that, due to the original fall of man from grace and God, chaos was the default position of the human race and that order came at a price, a price they were willing to pay, or at least a price that they were willing to urge others to pay. After all they were priests, and they were uncompromising in their insistence that clergy were properly exempt, or rather prohibited, from serving in the military or in any position that required them to shed blood.

In his advocacy of military service and martial virtues, Ambrose found vision and validation in the Hebrew Scriptures. Here he encountered the paradigms he needed to authorize him to write with enthusiasm of the "courage, which in war preserves one's country from the barbarians, or at home defends the weak, or comrades from robbers," adding that such courage is "full of justice."[6] Moses, Joshua, and David were among his preeminent exemplars of transparent faith and battlefield courage. He considered such courage or fortitude, as he preferred to call it, "a loftier virtue than the rest . . . for it prefers death to slavery and disgrace."[7] Furthermore, he argues, fortitude must never stand alone, as "fortitude without justice is the source of wickedness. For the stronger it is, the more ready is it to crush the weaker, whilst in matters of war one ought to see whether the war is just or unjust."[8] Ambrose saw two kinds of wars as unquestionably just: the first were holy wars declared by God, and the second were wars waged in defense of the state, to protect its borders, people, and property. Regarding the latter, his praise of public and especially military service was unstinting.

> It is considered . . . a glorious thing for each one at risk to himself to seek the quiet of all, and to think it far more thankworthy to have saved his country from destruction than to have kept danger from himself. We must think it a far more noble thing to labor for our country than to pass a quiet life at ease in the full enjoyment of leisure.[9]

What made possible Ambrose's riffs on the glories of war in the service of God or of God's most favored nation was his ability to bracket and bypass the gospel of peace broadcast in the New Testament, which so many Christian thinkers before him took to have abrogated the bellicosity of the Old Testament world.

6. Ambrose, *Duties of the Clergy,* I.27.129.
7. Ibid., I.35.176, I.41.211.
8. Ibid., I.35.176.
9. Ibid., III.3.23.

The key to Ambrose's freedom from the Sermon on the Mount, or the Last Discourse of Jesus in the Gospel of John, or any of the other sayings of Jesus that called for a life of nonviolence, was his appeal to, and interpretation of, Paul's pivotal axiom that "the letter kills, but the Spirit gives life" (2 Cor 3:6). Augustine, in his *Confessions*, tells how these words of Paul and their transformative effect on the teaching and preaching of Ambrose, provided the key to his own reading and acceptance of Scripture. "I was delighted," relates Augustine,

> to hear Ambrose in his sermons to the people saying, as if he were most carefully enunciating a principle of exegesis: "the letter kills, the spirit gives life." Those texts, which taken literally, seemed to contain perverse teaching he would expound spiritually, removing the mystical veil.[10]

However doubtful it may be that either Ambrose or Augustine understood the words of Paul and their implications precisely as Paul himself had when first writing them, they gladly embraced the radical freedom they found therein. Keen and opinionated intellects, like those of Ambrose and Augustine, were not to be yoked to a literal reading of the Bible, particularly when it affronted reason and contradicted firmly held truths and convictions.

What this meant regarding Christian military and civil service—service that entailed the exercise of violence and the shedding of blood—was that even the most explicitly pacific precepts of the gospels could be interiorized and made to mean something very different from what earlier Christians had taken them to mean. With the discretion to read practically any verse of Scripture as allegory, it was not long before the message of nonviolence, so central to Tertullian's and Origen's understanding of Christianity, became moot. Examples of this fact abound in the writings of Augustine, as when he sets out to interpret this familiar injunction of Jesus: "But I say to you, Do not resist an evildoer. But if anyone strikes you on the right cheek, turn the other also" (Matt 5:39; cf. Luke 6:29). Confronted with this and similar passages, Augustine proposed that we not "consider ourselves under bondage to the literal interpretation,"[11] arguing instead that Jesus never intended his words to deter or restrain his followers from the use of force, even lethal force, against evildoers. Instead, he writes, we should know that

10. Augustine, *Confessions* VI.4.6.
11. Augustine, *Letters*, 138.2.12 (*NPNF*).

> these precepts pertain rather to the inward disposition of the heart
> than to the actions which are done in the sight of men, requiring
> us, in the inmost heart, to cherish patience along with benevo-
> lence, but in the outward action to do that which seems most likely
> to benefit those whose good we ought to seek.[12]

Actions are one thing, and the intention or inward disposition that accom-
panies them is quite another. The former is what everyone sees, while the
latter is what God alone sees, and it is what God sees that matters.

Augustine made this crucial point quite dramatically when he commented on the act of *traditio,* more specifically the action of "handing over"
or "delivering up" Jesus to his crucifixion. "There was," he wrote,

> a "traditio" by the Father; there was a "traditio" by the Son; there
> was a "traditio" by Judas: the thing done is the same, but what is it
> that distinguishes the Father delivering up the Son, the Son deliv-
> ering up Himself, and Judas the disciple delivering up his Master?
> This: that the Father and the Son did it in love, but Judas did this in
> treacherous betrayal. . . . The diverse intention therefore makes the
> things done diverse. Though the thing be one, yet if we measure it
> by the diverse intentions, we find the one a thing to be loved, the
> other to be condemned; the one we find a thing to be glorified, the
> other to be detested. Such is the force of charity. See that it alone
> discriminates, it alone distinguishes the doings of men.[13]

There is no such literal thing, then, as an "act of love" or an "act of hate"—for
example, an intimate embrace or a lethal blow. Either might be performed
out of love or hate or any one of a number of diverse intents and inner
dispositions. It is the heart, the inner disposition of soul, that determines
the character of anything we do. And for the Christian, there is but one
disposition that surpasses all others and contains all that Jesus taught, and
lived, and was: Love. "God is Love" and "Love is God." These words were a
mantra for Augustine, and they are what he would have us consider before
we act, when we act, and when we look back and assess what we have done.
"See what we are insisting upon," he explains, "that the deeds of men are
only discerned by the root of charity. . . . Once for all, then, a precept is
given to thee: Love and do what thou wilt."[14]

12. Ibid., 138.2.13.

13. Augustine, *Ten Homilies,* 10.7.7.

14. Ibid., 10.7.8.

On the night before he died, in the account attributed to John the Apostle, Jesus left his disciples with one final instruction, the epitome of all that he had taught them: "I give you a new commandment, that you love one another. Just as I have loved you, you should also love one another" (John 13:34). While the early Christian church was inclined to take these words quite literally as, among others things, prohibiting Christian participation in war and capital punishment, Augustine saw in them no such restrictions. The Christian commandment of love, as Augustine understood it, does not altogether preclude such actions as killing, physically punishing, or even torturing others so as to make the world a safer, more just place, so long as these acts are guided by the right intention and performed in love, rather than in one or other dark personal passion, such as hatred, rage, or revenge.

Augustine considered the distinction and divide between the heart and the hand, between the inner disposition and the outward act, to be both grounded in Scripture and responsive to the necessities of life in a sinful world. He regarded the state, whether it be the pagan empire of Augustus or the Christian empire of Constantine, as a providential gift of God, a needed consolation in the fallen state of humanity. Without the heavy hand of a sovereign power to protect its people from enemies without and from criminals within, and to uphold some standard of justice, the human condition would be intolerable, as well as unconducive to the survival and spread of Christianity. "Surely, it is not without purpose," he wrote to Macedonius in 414,

> that we have the institution of the power of kings, the death penalty of the judge, the barbed hooks of the executioner, the weapons of the soldier, the right of punishment of the overlord, even the severity of the good father. All those things have their methods, their causes, their reasons, their practical benefits. While these are feared, the wicked are kept within bounds, and the good live more peacefully among the wicked.[15]

And the purpose he has in mind is not merely human purpose, but also divine purpose; for all that happens is seen and willed by God.

What all this means, for Augustine, with reference to the exercise of lethal force, is that not all killing is murder. "If to kill a man is homicide," we read in an early dialogue with his pupil Evodius, "it can sometimes be done without sin":

> When a soldier kills an enemy, or when a judge or an officer of the law puts a criminal to death, or when a weapon slips out of

15. Augustine, *Letters*, 153.6.16 (Parsons, 3:293).

someone's hand without his will or knowledge, the killing of a man does not seem to me to be a sin.[16]

What ultimately determines whether killing is evil, that is, sinful, is the intent and inner disposition of the killer. It is not the taking of life that is sinful. That act in itself is neutral and at times necessary, like sex. The moral problem with the sex act, we recall, is that it is all but impossible to perform without passion, that is, without erotic desire and blinding pleasure in which the pure intent to propagate becomes secondary or extraneous. Lovers are all too prone to come together out of a craving to delight each other and themselves rather than out of a biblical mandate to multiply. Of course, we might raise similar concerns regarding killing, particularly in war. It is no easy task to go to war and to engage in combat without passion, without hatred, rage, or revenge. And Augustine would agree with this, which points to why monks, nuns, and the clergy can never be asked or permitted to expose themselves to the heat of battle or the ardor of a lover's bed.

Violent death was, for Augustine, not a matter of ultimate concern, either for the one suffering it or for the one inflicting it. Death is a necessity faced by all, either sooner or later; and, measured against eternity, the difference between "sooner" and "later" is of even less concern. What truly matters is what never dies—the soul—and the state of the soul is in God's hands. "What is the evil in war?" asks Augustine:

Is it the death of some who will soon die in any case, that others may live in peaceful subjection? This is mere cowardly dislike, not any religious feeling. The real evils in war are love of violence, revengeful cruelty, fierce and implacable enmity, wild resistance, and the lust of power, and such like; and it is generally to punish these things, when force is required to inflict the punishment, that, in obedience to God or some lawful authority, good men undertake wars, when they find themselves in such a position as regards the conduct of human affairs, that right conduct requires them to act, or to make others act in this way.[17]

Killing, it seems, is not a moral issue. Rather, it is a simple necessity in our violent world, where peace and the common good are precarious and in need of enforcement and preservation. Violence can be good or it can be evil. The same act can be performed with a rightful intent and a pure heart, or may, instead, be undertaken with a wrongful intent and accompanied

16. Augustine, *On Free Will*, I.4.9.
17. Augustine, *Reply to Faustus*, 22.74.

by any of a number of dark passions that poison the soul. The difference between a killer and a murderer is not in what they do but in why and how they do it. This is not only the teaching and conviction of Augustine but also that of many, if not most, warriors in today's military. Shannon French, for years a professor of ethics at the United States Naval Academy, has reported how nearly without exception her midshipmen and -women students have insisted on a clear distinction between killers and murderers. "It is very important to them," she writes, "that I understand that while most warriors do *kill* people, they never *murder* anyone."[18] When asked to explain the difference between warriors, like themselves, trained to kill as agents of the state and simple murderers, they offered a range of suggestions, of which the following are representative:

- Murder is committed in cold blood, without a reason. A warrior should only kill in battle, when it is unavoidable.

- Murderers have no noble reason for their crimes.

- While a murderer often kills innocent or defenseless people, a warrior restricts his killing to willing combatants. He may stray, but that is an error, not the norm.

- A murderer is someone who kills and enjoys it. That is not a warrior.

- A murderer is one who usually kills innocent, unarmed people, while a warrior has honor in battle and does not take advantage of the weak.

- A murderer murders out of hate. A warrior does not. He knows how to control his anger.

- A warrior is not a murderer because a warrior has a code that he lives by which is influenced by morals that must be justified.

- Warriors fight other warriors. Therefore they kill rather than murder.

- Murder lacks any implication of honor or ethics, but rather calls to mind ruthlessness and disregard for human life.

- A murderer kills for gain, or out of anger. He does not allow victims a fair fight.

- The term *murder* represents an act done with malice. Warriors kill people in an honorable way.

- A murderer has no honor.[19]

18. French, *Code of the Warrior*, 20.
19. Ibid.

The crucial differentiating factors noted by these men and women, warriors-in-training, can be distilled into several categories: intent, inner disposition, authorization, and victims. Warriors, or state-deputized killers, must have a noble or just cause and must purge themselves of such compromising and corrupting passions and emotions as anger, hatred, greed, malice, or enjoyment. Augustine, as we have seen, is in full accord with such assertions. Furthermore, warriors direct their violence at and kill other warriors, not innocent noncombatants. Augustine, for his part, was less concerned with this distinction, recognizing that the killing of civilians was a necessary foregone conclusion in war, something he saw as unfortunate but not so evil as to make the warrior into a murderer.

One of the most curious and, at first glance, confounding assertions of both Ambrose and Augustine regarding the legitimate exercise of lethal force against others, was their unconditional condemnation of personal self-defense. This was, as they saw it, always a sin, always evil. Killing in defense of the state was one thing, and killing to defend one's own life or property was something very different. "As to killing others in order to defend one's own life," Augustine wrote in 398,

> I do not approve of this, unless one happens to be a soldier or public functionary acting, not for himself, but in defense of others or of the city in which he resides, if he acts according to the commission lawfully given him, and in the manner becoming his office.[20]

Augustine's position on self-defense may well have been influenced and shaped by his revered mentor, Ambrose, who stated his position in this manner:

> I do not think that a Christian, a just and a wise man, ought to save his own life by the death of another; just as when he meets with an armed robber he cannot return his blows, lest in defending his life he should stain his love toward his neighbour. The verdict on this is plain and clear in the books of the Gospel. "Put up thy sword, for every one that taketh the sword shall perish with the sword." What robber is more hateful than the persecutor who came to kill Christ? But Christ would not be defended from the wounds of the persecutor, for He willed to heal all by His wounds.[21]

20. Augustine, *Letters*, 47.5 (*NPNF*).
21. Ambrose, *Duties of the Clergy*, III.4.27.

The reappearance of the biblical and early Christian case for pacifism may well seem startling in this of all instances; for to all but the most rigorous and uncompromising pacifists, self-defense often represents the single, clearest exception to the divine command not to kill.

There are, I believe, two patent principles governing the denunciation of self-defense by Ambrose and Augustine. The first is that, for them, killing must be authorized by a sovereign authority. Otherwise it is murder and truly sinful. The true sovereign, of course, is God, the Creator and Savior of the world. The wars of the Old Testament, so often and enthusiastically cited by Ambrose and Augustine, were manifestly authorized by God, and so the men that waged them were saints rather than sinners, even when they slaughtered and pillaged the enemy, combatants and noncombatants alike. The other sovereign authority is the state, which is not God but which they believed to represent an extension of the divine imperium, "for there is no authority except from God, and those authorities that exist have been instituted by God" (Rom 13:1). Ambrose celebrated the Christian empire of Constantine and his successors as coming all the more directly from God, but Augustine was more circumspect here. Regardless, both men acknowledged that there were good rulers and regimes and bad ones, and that even good rulers could make bad decisions. None of this deeply mattered, however, when it came to the authorization of violence. Whether a war, or for that matter a judicial sentence, was just or unjust weighed on the conscience of the sovereign or judge, not on that of the soldier and the executioner, who must concern themselves only with following the orders given them and doing so with the right intent and inner disposition.

In his determination to draw a sharp line between self-defense and defense of the state, and to condemn the one while condoning the other, Augustine added an additional, rather peculiar supporting argument. He pointed out, citing Cicero, that

> "death is not natural to a republic as to a man, to whom death is not only necessary, but often even desirable. But when a state is destroyed, obliterated, annihilated, it is as if (to compare great things with small) this whole world perished and collapsed" . . . For death, as he [Cicero] says, is no punishment to individuals, but rather delivers them from all other punishments, but it is a punishment to the state.[22]

---

22. Augustine, *City of God*, 22.6.

Apart from the fact that many of the "individuals" for whom Augustine here presumes to speak might dissent from the opinion that the imposition of death is no punishment, it seems gratuitous to claim that death is more natural to the individual than to the state. Augustine knew enough history to have witnessed the phenomenal fact that states rise and fall as surely as do human beings. Admittedly, their respective life spans differ significantly, but to exempt republics from the evanescence of all existence is a stretch. And to confirm Cicero's claim that "when a state is destroyed . . . it is as if this whole world perished and collapsed" is even more of a stretch. The collapse of more than one state in antiquity and since has brought shouts of relief and joy rather than shrieks of despair. In fact, the Roman Empire was responsible for any number of such collapses and was on the verge of experiencing its own.

The core of Augustine's argument against self-defense nevertheless rested on the fact that the person who kills in self-defense acts without any authorization from God or country. To make matters worse, it was all but inconceivable to Ambrose and Augustine that such an act could possibly be prompted and accompanied by a right intent and inner disposition of soul. In their eyes, killing to save one's own skin betrays an inordinate, self-ish attachment to incarnate existence and too little attention to the divine commands not to kill and to love others as much as oneself. Furthermore, how could anyone dispassionately kill an attacker? Would not fear, anger, and rage surge up and take possession of the soul; and how would anyone avoid feelings of relief and satisfaction when, at the end of the struggle, the assailant and not oneself lies dead? Far better, they argue, not to sin in order to prolong a life that is inevitably brief, but rather to die like Christ, a lamb slain without resistance, and to meet one's Maker and Redeemer without the mark of Cain stamped on one's forehead.

There are many surprising gaps and silences in the writings of Augustine—surprising in part because the corpus of his extant works numbers well over a hundred (116 to be exact), but more surprising because they cry out even today for some response from him. One of these is his apparent assumption that killing in war could be dispassionate, free of anger, hatred, rage, revenge, and thrill. The fact that he himself never served in the military nor shed blood is not enough to excuse him from learning something from those who did or from at least exercising his imagination to put himself in their place. His own extensive sexual experience as a young man had moderated his views on the evils of pleasurable sex, having learned all too well on his own that a certain degree of erotic delight was unavoidable and thus pardonable. Perhaps he also realized all too well that dispassionate warcraft was an impossible fiction and so, as a result, was the line he had drawn between killing and murder. Yet, if his theory of war without sin was a fiction it was a convenient one. In reading his massive masterwork, *The City of God*, we come to appreciate how bleak was his vision of this life in the City of Man, how dangerous and depraved our condition, how desperately in need of some sources of order and earthly peace, what he called the "Peace of Babylon." Recalling that in the year 476, as he lay on his deathbed and recited the penitential psalms, the Vandals were laying siege to his own city of Hippo, may help us to put in some perspective his having provided the foundation and footprint for an enduring Christian endorsement of violence for the sake of order, security, and even orthodoxy.

A second disturbing hiatus in Augustine's widely scattered comments on military and judicial violence may be seen in his never having addressed the problem of personal conscience, specifically the conscience of a soldier or executioner confronting a lethal command that he or she considers to be unjust or evil. Granted, he did foresee the possibility that a legitimate authority might order a soldier to commit a sacrilegious or idolatrous act and stated that such an order should not be obeyed.[23] It seems never to have occurred to Augustine, however, that in war a soldier might be given an order that he could not in good conscience obey. But how is that possible? It is more likely that he chose not to raise the issue but to leave it to others to deal with. As a priest and bishop it was not a situation he would ever personally be required to face. On one occasion, however, a friend and general named Boniface apparently brought to him his concerns over the life he had chosen, expressing a desire to leave the army and enter a monastery. Augustine, in response, reassured him that, like David, he was serving God in his military service and thus dissuaded him from abandoning it. "Do not think," wrote Augustine, "that it is impossible for any one to please God while engaged in active military service."[24] Augustine went on to urge Boniface to wage war always for the sake of peace, and so to be numbered among the peacemakers. "Think, then, of this first of all," he goes on, "when you are arming for the battle, that even your bodily strength is a gift of God."[25] Counsel such as this is as commonplace today as then, particularly coming from the mouths of clergy in uniform, designated to

23. See Augustine, *Expositions*, 125.7.
24. Augustine, *Letters*, 189.4 (*NPNF*).
25. Ibid., 189.6.

serve the spiritual needs of warriors while not detracting from their battle-readiness, their "battlemind."

Similar counsel appears to have been foreseen and expected from the empire's first formal military chaplains—Christian bishops invited by Constantine to accompany his legions on their expeditions. Eusebius, in his *The Life of Constantine the Great*, relates how Constantine went about summoning bishops to his side and what his expectations of them included:

> It is also worthy of record that about the time of which I am at present writing, the emperor, having heard of an insurrection of some barbarians in the East, observed that the conquest of this enemy was still in store for him, and resolved on an expedition against the Persians. Accordingly he proceeded at once to put his forces in motion, at the same time communicating his intended march to the bishops who happened to be at his court, some of whom he judged it right to take with him as companions, and as needful coadjutors in the service of God. They, on the other hand, cheerfully declared their willingness to follow in his train, disclaiming any desire to leave him, and engaging to battle with and for him by supplication to God on his behalf. Full of joy at this answer to his request, he unfolded to them his projected line of march; after which he caused a tent of great splendor, representing in shape the figure of a church, to be prepared for his own use in the approaching war. In this he intended to unite with the bishops in offering prayers to the God from whom all victory proceeds.[26]

In reading Eusebius' account we should not pass over lightly his referring to the bishops as his "needful coadjutors" nor the fact that he refers to his war against Persian barbarians as the "service of God." The barbarians, as Ambrose later confirmed, were the empire's and the church's natural enemies, and defense of the empire amounted to defense of the faith. "The larger implicit claim seems to be that while Roman wars fought against barbarians are just," writes Lieutenant Colonel John Mark Mattox, "any war initiated by the barbarians is unjust."[27] Christian-Roman "exceptionalism" will be the first of countless exceptionalisms claimed by future states and religions invoking just war theory and claiming that by definition any war they wage is just and any war waged against them is unjust.

26. Eusebius, *Life of Constantine*, IV.56.
27. Mattox, *Saint Augustine*, 20.

And so Constantine went to war with bishops at his side and with the sign of the cross as a "triumphant charm" before him. Eusebius tells us how the emperor

> caused the sign of the salutary trophy [the sign of the cross] to be impressed on the very shields of his soldiers; and commanded that his embattled forces should be preceded in their march, not by golden images, as heretofore, but only by the standard of the cross. . . . Indeed, wherever this appeared, the enemy soon fled before his victorious troops. And the emperor perceiving this, whenever he saw any part of his forces hard pressed, gave orders that the salutary trophy should be moved in that direction, like some triumphant charm against disasters: at which the combatants were divinely inspired, as it were, with fresh strength and courage, and immediate victory was the result.[28]

There is no mistaking the fact that in the fourth and fifth centuries the Lamb of God was being rapidly redesigned into the Lord of Hosts. The seed of holy war had been sown and was already taking root in welcoming soil. The imperial legions were now the agents of God, the enforcers of his will, the devouring flame of his wrath. Just how far this conceit could and would be taken was showcased in the year 388 when Ambrose the Bishop intervened to restrain the Emperor Theodosius from punishing a Christian community in Callinicum for burning down a Jewish synagogue. Ambrose assembled a number of arguments to make his case, concluding that "there is, then, no adequate cause for such a commotion, that the people should be so severely punished for the burning of a building, and much less since it is the burning of a synagogue, a home of unbelief, a house of impiety, a receptacle of folly, which God Himself has condemned."[29] For centuries the early Christian church had prayed for and come to expect religious tolerance within a pagan empire, and for the most part they had been granted it. Now, when the empire was theirs, they forgot all that. They forgot as well the second greatest commandment given them by their Lord and Savior, to love their neighbor as they loved themselves (Matt 22:36–39; Mark 12:28–31; Luke 10:27). He must have meant their Christian neighbor.

By the close of the fourth century, if not earlier, Christians had only two valid options for weighing the morality of military service and the killing that it entailed: pacifism and the just war theory. The latter represented

28. Eusebius, *Life of Constantine*, IV.21, II.7
29. Ambrose, *Letters*, 40.14.

the official position of the church and would continue to do so far into the future (down to the moment when I am writing this sentence). The former position, the total renunciation of all bloodshed, would remain the personal prerogative of the church's "first estate"—monks, nuns, and clergy—as well as the personal choice of a relative handful of men and women who were more convinced by the gospels than they were by the theology of Ambrose, Augustine, Eusebius, and others. One such pacifist was Saint Martin, a legionnaire in the army of Julian in the year 356. After contributing to a decisive Roman victory, Martin, to the astonishment and anger of his commander, refused his "donative" or due reward and, instead, chose this moment to declare, "Up to the present I have served in your army; permit me now to be a soldier of Christ; it is not right for me to fight."[30] Then, to prove that his refusal to fight was a matter of conscience and not cowardice, he pledged himself in the next day's battle to march in the front lines "without shield or helmet but protected by the sign of the cross."[31] As it happened, there was to be no battle the next day, as the enemy chose instead to surrender without a fight, an event in which Martin's biographer, Sulpitius Severus, saw the miraculous hand of God. In addition to the isolated conscientious objector like Martin, there was the lone voice of the occasional bishop and theologian who supported his position, but these types were increasingly marginal figures in a triumphal church.

Before we leave the church of late antiquity and proceed into the Middle Ages, there is one more voice to which we need to listen, and that is the muted voice of uneasiness and uncertainty perceptible in a church that has for all practical purposes embraced the not very limiting policy and practice of just war—not very limiting because the wars that it supported were deemed just by definition. We listen here to a letter written by Saint Basil the Great of Caesarea to his friend Amphilochius of Iconium, a fourth-century bishop who before he took up his episcopal duties in Cappadocia had been first a lawyer and later a monk:

> Homicide in war is not reckoned by our Fathers as homicide; I presume from their wish to make concession to men fighting on behalf of chastity and true religion. Perhaps, however, it is well to counsel that those whose hands are not clean only abstain from communion for three years.[32]

30. "Life of St. Martin," 4, cited in Swift, *Early Fathers*, 151.
31. Ibid.
32. Basil, *Letters*, 188.XIII.

The disconnect in these words that on the face of it declare that homicide in war is not homicide may be seen first in the use of the word "concession" to describe this declaration. The ability to kill without it's being called homicide comes to the soldier as a special dispensation or waiver. But not without a catch. Those who kill in war are to be counseled to abstain from communion for three years. In a word, they are to be temporarily "excommunicated." Presumably because they are stained, polluted, corrupted. They need to perform at least this penance: to remove themselves from the table of the Lord and the liturgical company of fellow Christians. And all this from a bishop and saint who wrote personally to a soldier these words of approval and blessing:

> I count no blessing greater than the knowledge of your excellency, which has been permitted me by our good Lord's mercy. I have learnt to know one who proves that even in a soldier's life it is possible to preserve the perfection of love to God, and that we must mark a Christian not by the style of his dress, but by the disposition of his soul. It was a great delight to me to meet you; and now, whenever I remember you, I feel very glad. Play the man; be strong; strive to nourish and multiply love to God, that there may be given you by Him yet greater boons of blessing.[33]

Basil, like the church that he eminently represents in the fourth century, has learned to speak with two tongues regarding and to Christian men in uniform. They are encouraged to enlist and go off to war with a clear conscience, marching behind the standard of Christ with courage and resolve, but at the same time to realize that their shedding of blood, while not sinful, renders them unclean and thus unworthy to approach the altar of the same Lord who led them into battle. The church, or at least some prominent voices in the church, seemed to suffer from a pacifist lump in their throat, a lump that in no way kept them from affirming the theory of just war and its concomitant distinction between killing and murder, but in every way kept them from ever putting on a uniform or taking up a weapon themselves. We may conclude from this that the Christian mind on military service was not yet made up.

33. Ibid., 106.

6

Medieval Christianity

Warriors and Monks

ROMULUS AUGUSTUS, THE LAST emperor of Rome, had a twenty-four-karat name. Romulus was, of course, Rome's legendary founder and first king, while Augustus created its empire. Romulus Augustus, however, was related to neither of these and managed only to preside over Rome's demise. So minor a figure was he and so loose his grip on power that his removal more closely resembled an early retirement than a revolution. Unlike so many other less fortunate, fallen sovereigns, he kept his head as well as an annual pension and lived out his days in palatial comfort. When placed in power by his father, Romulus had been a mere teenager, with a penchant for poetry, and his reign had lasted only months. The year was 476 and Simplicius was bishop of Rome, the forty-seventh pope in the line of Saint Peter.

As the lights went out in the Old Rome, signaling the start of the so-called Dark Ages, countless candles still burned in the churches of the New Rome, the Ecclesia Catholica, an emerging empire of a different sort, but an empire nonetheless. The ascendant Roman Catholic Church was on an ambitious trajectory of its own. In the ensuing centuries it would become the center of Western Christendom, whose borders would reach far beyond those of the Roman Empire at its zenith. It defined rather than defied the *saeculum*, the earthly order. With regard to internal matters of doctrine and discipline, papal hegemony could be summed up in the saying: *Roma locuta*

86

est, casa finita est, or "Rome has spoken. Case closed." But the church did not limit itself to "internal matters." In fact it never had, not since it became both legal and privileged under Constantine. Already in 390, Ambrose, bishop of Milan, had presumed to confront face to face the last ruler of an undivided Roman Empire, Theodosius the Great, and to bar his entrance into the church where Ambrose was celebrating the Mass, on the grounds that Theodosius—provoked by sedition in Macedonia—had slaughtered over seven thousand people in the city of Thessalonica, without a trial. In response, Theodosius did penance and enacted a new law, dictated to him by Ambrose, that would limit the emperor's power to execute his people at will, without a proper trial and period of review. Theodoret's fifth-century account of this episode concludes with this glimpse into the balance or imbalance of power between the emperor and the bishop:

> Now the very faithful emperor came boldly within the holy temple but did not pray to his Lord standing, or even on his knees, but lying prone upon the ground he uttered David's cry, "My soul cleaveth unto the dust, quicken thou me according to thy word." He plucked out his hair; he smote his head; he besprinkled the ground with drops of tears and prayed for pardon. When the time came for him to bring his oblations to the holy table, weeping all the while he stood up and approached the sanctuary. After making his offering, as he was wont, he remained within at the rail, but once more the great Ambrosius kept not silence and taught him the distinction of places. First he asked him if he wanted anything; and when the emperor said that he was waiting for participation in the divine mysteries, Ambrose sent word to him by the chief deacon and said, "The inner place, sir, is open only to priests; to all the rest it is inaccessible; go out and stand where others stand; purple can make emperors, but not priests."[1]

"Purple can make emperors, but not priests." These words came as a line in the sand to the emperor, pointing out to him his place, his subordinate place. In the eyes of the church, which is to say in the eyes of God, he is a layman, a member of the second estate, one of the countless *kosmikoi* or "men of the world," whose relation to God and salvation are mediated to them by the clergy, the bishops, and ultimately the pope, the successor of Peter. This is not to say that priests, of whatever rank, were not often, to all appearances, as worldly as the laity. Rather, it was to claim that "the ordained" and "the consecrated" were supernaturally endowed with powers

1. Theodoret, *Ecclesisastical History*, V.17. See also Ambrose, *Letters*, 51.

and prerogatives that placed them apart from, and elevated them above, other men, not by virtue of who they were but by virtue of what they had become, the supernaturally empowered agents of God. The ancient *cursus honorum*, the traditional ladder of advancement within the Roman Empire's political bureaucracy, was replaced by the ecclesiastical sequence of Holy Orders, an ascending series of offices and powers, each with its own sacramental ritual of ordination or consecration.

The sharp line drawn—might we even say the deep trench dug—by Ambrose between clergy and laity in fact marked a departure from the earlier understanding of the Christian priesthood. During the first few centuries of Christianity, priests were chosen ad hoc, as it were, to serve the evolving needs of Christian cult. Ecclesiae or worshipping communities chose from their own number those who would preside over the offering of the gifts, the *thusia* or sacrifice of the Mass, and the baptism of neophytes. In the words of Tertullian,

> Are not even we, the laity, priests? It is written: "A kingdom also, and priests to His God and Father, hath He made us." It is the authority of the Church, and the honour which has acquired sanctity through the joint session of the ordained, which has established the difference between the ordained and the laity. Accordingly, where there is no joint session of the ecclesiastical ordained, you offer, and baptize, and are priest, alone for yourself. But where three are, a church is, albeit they be laity. For each individual lives by his own faith, nor is there exception of persons with God; since it is not hearers of the law who are justified by the Lord, but doers, according to what the apostle withal says. Therefore, if you have the right of a priest in your own person, in cases of necessity, it behooves you to have likewise the discipline of a priest whenever it may be necessary to have the right of a priest.[2]

In other words, the power and authority of an ordained priest or a consecrated bishop are not his own but belong to and are derived from the authority of the church, the *ecclesia*, the assembly of the faithful. In such an assembly—wherever two or three are gathered in Christ's name—any layman among them can, in the absence of an "official" ordained priest and with the consent of those assembled, serve as priest and do what a priest does. "Official" priests and bishops owe their ordination and office to the unanimous election by the community. This was how both Ambrose and

2. Tertullian, *Exhortation to Chastity*, VII. Translation slightly modernized for clarity.

Augustine, and those before them, rose to the priesthood—by acclamation. Even as late as the High Middle Ages we see the same principle being asserted in that "a bishop must be chosen *ab omni populo* [by all the people] and ordained *consentibus omnibus* [with the consent of all]."[3]

What this meant in the early church, prior to Ambrose and Augustine, was that even an official, ordained priest—deposed or severed from the assembly by apostasy, heresy, schism, or a sinful life—forfeits his priesthood together with all of its powers. His priesthood, in such an instance, comes to nothing. In truth it was never "his" in the first place. Just as in a modern democracy an impeached president is an ordinary citizen, so in ancient Christianity a deposed priest was an ordinary layman. Sometime in the late fourth century, however, this all began to change. In a church infected with schism and heresy and divided against itself, there were those who claimed that sacraments performed by heretical, schismatic, or otherwise unworthy priests were invalid. Some even argued that this invalidation of priestly powers and actions was retroactive, in other words that sacraments previously performed by a once proper priest, now no longer in good standing, were "undone," requiring, for example, that once-baptized Christians be rebaptized or that once-ordained priests be reordained.[4] Clearly, this threatened the church with chaotic insecurity and undermined the Christian priesthood precisely at that point in the church's development when those like Ambrose, Augustine, and Eusebius wished to elevate that priesthood to an otherworldly status it had never previously enjoyed.

The new, transformative understanding of Christian priesthood that emerged and began to take hold in the Western church at the turn of the fourth to the fifth century conferred upon priests at ordination a *dominicus character indelebilis*, complete with accompanying supernatural powers resembling those of Jesus the Wonderworker, the very powers promised to Peter in these words: "I will give you the keys of the kingdom of heaven, and whatever you bind on earth will be bound in heaven, and whatever you loose on earth will be loosed in heaven" (Matt 16:19). Once a priest, always a priest—forever, no matter what. An ordained priest may lose his faith, lose his soul, lose his mind, but he can do nothing to lose his priesthood. Nor can it be taken from him. Furthermore, when performing his most

3. Campenhausen, *Tradition*, 221.

4. For example, the Council of Nicaea (325 CE) spoke to the need for re-baptism or re-ordination in certain circumstances where those previously baptized or ordained had embraced schism or heresy. Later, in 451 CE, the Council of Chalcedon addressed conditions under which an ordination should be revoked or declared null after the fact.

sacred duties, the administration of the sacraments—baptizing, forgiving sins, celebrating the Eucharist, ordaining other priests, and so on—his motives, his inner disposition, the state of his soul, all count for nothing regarding the validity and effectiveness of his ritual acts. The formula developed in the twelfth century to designate the autonomic effectiveness of a priest's sacramental actions was *ex opere operato*, meaning that the effect proceeds from the work or act (*opus*) having been performed. When the prescribed act is done and the prescribed words are uttered, the sacrament is perfectly complete and irreversible. Sins forgiven by a sinner and sins forgiven by a saint are equally forgiven. Bread and wine over which the words of consecration have been spoken by a priest becomes the body and blood of Christ, whether the priest has performed this rite to nourish the hungry souls of the faithful or to provide impious souls with an opportunity for desecration. Not without reason, the powers of this new priesthood have been compared with magic and the priest himself seen as a Christian magus.

While the primary impetus behind this radical reconsideration of the Catholic priesthood may have been concern for the security of the sacraments and the peace of mind of the faithful, it also served to elevate priests to new heights in the firmament. The authority of priests and of their high priest, the Bishop of Rome, was seen to trump that of emperors and kings, who for all their thrones and trappings were mere laity. All in good time, the imperial church rose and asserted itself. Already in the late fifth century, Pope Gelasius wrote to Emperor Anastasius to remind him of his penultimate place in the earthly scheme:

> There are two powers, august Emperor, by which this world is chiefly ruled, namely, the sacred authority of the priests and the royal power. Of these that of the priests is the more weighty. . . . You are also aware, dear son, that while you are permitted honorably to rule over human kind, yet in things divine you bow your head humbly before the leaders of the clergy and await from their hands the means of your salvation.[5]

The church, however, eventually extended its primacy beyond "things divine" and claimed what today is called "full-spectrum dominance." A high-water mark in the imperial pretensions of the church may surely be found in the papal bull titled *Unam Sanctam*, promulgated by Pope Boniface VIII on November 18, 1302. In this remarkable document aimed at

5. Robinson, *Readings*, I.72.

King Philip the Fair of France, Boniface, invoking Luke 22:38, recalled the two swords proffered to Jesus on the night of his death, to which Jesus replied, "It is enough." He then went on to state that only the spiritual sword is wielded *by* the church, while the material sword is wielded *for* the church (by kings and their armies) at her discretion and will. Boniface left no room here for any lingering doubt regarding the subordination of all secular authority and power to that of the church, vested in the person of the pope, when he concluded his missive with these words: "Furthermore, we declare, state, define and pronounce that it is altogether necessary to salvation for every human creature to be subject to the Roman Pontiff."[6]

In fact, Boniface, in his confrontation with Philip, was only reminding the king of claims asserted centuries earlier by the church. The *Dictatus Papae* or "Dictates of the Pope," dating from the eleventh century and sometimes attributed to Pope Gregory VII, comprises a list of twenty-seven assumed principles or prerogatives of the papacy. These include the claim that the pope alone may use the imperial insignia and that all princes shall kiss his feet. Further, he asserts his right to depose emperors and to dissolve the bond between a king and his subjects. All sentences passed by him are binding and irrevocable, except by himself, and he is immune from judgment, not only by men but also by God, for his sanctity is guaranteed beyond doubt by the merits of Saint Peter, the first pope. It is indeed doubtful that even Ambrose, when he reminded his emperor that "purple can make emperors, but not priests," imagined just how far his words would someday be taken.

Returning now to the central focus and narrative of this book, it surely goes without saying that the imperial church of the early and High Middle Ages was no pacifist church. It continued to condone and not infrequently to call for the exercise of violence by the secular powers to whom the material sword was entrusted. At first and for the most part the church's first estate—those in Holy Orders or under sacred vows—left the killing to the laity and thus kept its hands clean. Its soul was another matter. It may be that the primary intent of the theory and rules of just war suggested by Augustine and developed by Aquinas was to limit rather than to legitimize lethal force, but that was hardly their primary effect. Sometimes to open a pinhole is to unleash a flood, particularly when the force to be controlled is immeasurably greater than the barriers placed in its path. Once again we must focus on the church's insistence that it

6. Bettenson, *Documents*, 161.

is the intent or intended consequence of an action that defines it. This philosophical doctrine, as we have already seen, was Christianity's key to legitimizing both lovemaking and warmaking. "For as in the Old Testament the outward works are observed," confirmed the Venerable Bede in the eighth century, "so in the New Testament, that which is outwardly done is not so diligently regarded as that which is inwardly thought."[7] As a result, "lawful commerce" or legitimate sex "must be for the sake of children"[8] not pleasure, though pleasure is unavoidable. Similarly, lawful killing must be for the sake of justice or a better peace, not rage or revenge. In either case, what must be avoided is passion, the disturbance of mind and soul, for "only the calm mind can rest in the light of contemplation."[9] Augustine, in his *City of God*, had mused on what prelapsarian sex must have been like in paradise, imagining that it would be an act entirely under the control of reason and will. Erection would be as voluntary as the lifting of one's arm and the love act itself equally so. Love-making, like the sipping of fine wine, would look nothing like the mad mayhem of later love, beyond the primordial garden. By extension, killing, though never practiced in paradise, should approximate the calm, calculated deliberation and control of a dancer—ballroom not mosh pit. Think killer-drone pilot and the right image might come to mind.

As it happens, we owe to Peter Abelard, the great and notorious French medieval Scholastic philosopher and theologian, the most acute exposition of the primacy of intent in determining and defining our deeds. In his ethical treatise titled *Know Yourself*, Abelard insists that all sin lies exclusively in the mind's consent to evil. The actual doing of the deed is irrelevant. The commission of a sinful act adds nothing to the guilt of a sinner, any more than the non-commission of a sinful act diminishes that guilt. Consent is an inward act and must be both conscious and willful. "God alone," writes Abelard, "pays attention not so much to the deeds that are done as to the mind with which they are done [and] is truly thinking about the guilt in our intention":

> Thus he is called the tester of the heart and the reins, and is said to see in darkness. For where no one sees, there he sees most of all, because in punishing sin he doesn't pay attention to the deed but

7. Bede, *Ecclesiastical History*, I.27.
8. Ibid.
9. Ibid.

to the mind, just as conversely we don't pay attention to the mind
that we don't see but to the deed we know.[10]

Presumably Abelard—castrated for his deeds not his desires—spoke from
experience here. It was only when his dalliances with Heloise were brought
to light that he was made to pay the price for them; for men do not see in
darkness nor avenge what happens there. But, we might wonder and ask,
are we not men? Ought we to imitate God and attend only to what the heart
intends and not to what the hand does? Abelard, like Augustine before him,
argues that two men can go to war and take life or go to bed and make
life. To an outward observer, their actions are identical, but to a discerner
of souls the one has sinned and deserves damnation while the other has
done right and deserves merit. The body count, dead or alive, apparently
doesn't deeply matter—not to God. But does it matter to us? Abelard seems
to acknowledge that it does.

Consequences—the visible, tangible outcome of our deeds—clearly
must be taken somehow into account. They obviously matter to people,
and even philosophers and theologians are people. This fact called for a
convenient distinction to be made between two kinds of consequences:
intended consequences and unintended consequences. Not surprisingly, it
is intended consequences that are said to truly matter. This means that as
a Christian layperson I can have sex without sin if the outcome I intend is
a son or a daughter. The pleasure I cannot help but enjoy in the process is
foreseen but unintended. A similar argument was employed by Thomas
Aquinas to overturn the earlier Ambrosian/Augustinian prohibition on
violent self-defense.[11] To ward off a threat to my life and so to preserve my
personal existence is, as Aquinas saw it, a self-evidently legitimate goal or
intent, and if I keep that foremost in my mind as I remove that threat, the
dead body that may soon lie in my doorway or at my feet represents an
unintended consequence of my will to live another day. This is the same
reasoning that today allows the Catholic Church on the one hand to condemn abortion, and on the other hand to approve the hysterectomy of a
pregnant woman suffering from uterine cancer. The foreseen certainty that
this procedure will terminate the woman's fetus does not constitute intent
to do so. The resulting "abortion" is an unintended consequence and, as
such, is a matter of no moral concern.

10. Abelard, *Ethical Writings*, I.84.

11. For Thomas Aquinas' discussion of the doctrine of double effect as applied to
self-defense, see *Summa Theologica* (II-II, Qu. 64, Art. 7).

The moral primacy of intent and what came to be known as the principle of double effect are, admittedly, pinholes—at first more or less harmless and surely compassionate. But through frequent use pinholes easily become loopholes, and exceptions can replace rules. Not all that many people today will begrudge lovers a little delight as they find their way to becoming parents, nor begrudge a woman the right to life-saving procedures even if it means losing the child in her womb. But the principle of double effect no longer stops there. In fact it never did. There is also the sniper firing all too effectively on U.S. troops from an apartment complex in Baghdad. To save lives, Army lives, he must be neutralized, and calling in an air strike is the quickest and surest way to accomplish that. Minutes later, the sniper's fire ceases, and the building that gave him cover is a smoldering pile. The other nameless lives lost in the action are its "other effect," the unintended, though foreseen, consequence of the destruction aimed at and intended for only one man. As we know, solitary air strikes can easily become bombing campaigns, taking not tens but millions of lives; but if the primary intention is to end war and make peace, then it would seem that all hands are clean and all consciences clear.

It takes little imagination or critical acuity to see that the principle of double effect and the immunizing primacy of personal intent are dangerous enablers for anyone without eyes wide open and without a moral compass in hand. Defining an intention as "an interior act of the mind that could be produced at will . . . and as all important . . . in determining the goodness or badness of an action," argued Oxford philosopher Elizabeth Anscombe, "is a marvelous way . . . of making any action lawful. You only had to 'direct your intention' in a suitable way."[12] Going on to address the related principle of double effect, Anscombe points out harshly but fairly that

> This same doctrine is used to prevent any doubts about the obliteration bombing of a city. The devout Catholic bomber secures by a "direction of intention" that any shedding of innocent blood that occurs is "accidental." I know a Catholic boy who was puzzled at being told by his schoolmaster that it was an accident that the people of Hiroshima and Nagasaki were there to be killed; in fact, however absurd it seems, such thoughts are common among priests who know that they are forbidden by the divine law to justify the direct killing of the innocent. It is nonsense to pretend

12. Anscombe, "War and Murder," 58.

that you do not intend to do what is the means you take to your chosen end.[13]

Whether it is fair to number Ambrose, Augustine, or Aquinas among such priests as Anscombe describes above remains, I would suggest, an open question at this point. Their primary intent, I believe and have already said, was to limit rather than to license violence, which they saw as inevitable and necessary; so any final assessment of their writings on war will likely depend on just how much weight should be given to their original intent and how much to their long-term effect.

Thomas Aquinas, to whom tradition has awarded the title "Angelic Doctor," represents the pinnacle of medieval scholastic theology. Despite the fact that only several months before his death Thomas is reported as having summed up his work with the words *mihi videtur ut palea* ("it seems to me as straw"),[14] his systematic rendering of Christian doctrine has been the measure of Roman Catholic Orthodoxy for nearly nine hundred years. As recently as 1960, Pope John XXIII reaffirmed the Catholic Church's unique and unequivocal adoption of the theological teachings of Thomas Aquinas as its own, stating that the writings of this revered Doctor of the church were in full accord with the truth of reason, the tradition of the Holy Fathers, and the revelation of Holy Scripture. What's more, the foundational character of Thomistic teaching is nowhere more evident than in his doctrine of just warfare. Virtually every later theory and argument regarding the determination of just war and the legislation of the rules of war has built upon what Thomas wrote on the subject in the second half of the thirteenth century. That said, the slice of his *Summa Theologica* allotted to the question of war is disconcertingly brief, even cursory.[15]

Thomas' answer to the question whether it is always sinful to wage war is characteristically precise and direct: "In order for a war to be just, three things are necessary." He then proceeds to list the three conditions he has in mind: (1) declaration of war by a legitimate sovereign authority; (2) for the sake of a just cause, such as avenging a wrong done or recovering what was unjustly taken; and (3) always with a right intention. Here, to elucidate what he means by a right intention, he quotes from Augustine and reminds the reader that war must be for the sake of peace, punishing evil, and uplifting the good. By contrast he condemns, again in words on

13. Ibid., 59.

14. McBride, *Development and Meaning*, 131.

15. Thomas Aquinas, *Summa Theologica*, II-II, Qu. 40.

loan from Augustine, "the passion for inflicting harm, the cruel thirst for vengeance, an unpacific and relentless spirit, the fever of revolt, the lust of power."[16] Thomas then goes on to respond to a few presumably hot-button questions at the time concerning the proper conduct of a just war, such as whether it is sinful for bishops and clergy to fight in war, whether it is right to lay ambushes, and whether war may be waged on designated holy days. His disapproval of combatant clergy and bloodshed on the Sabbath and holy days comes as no surprise, nor does his acceptance of ambushes as a fact of war. What is significant in these few and brief addenda to his definition of a just war is the fact that he acknowledges here that how a war is conducted can also be a matter of moral concern. There is no denying, however, that Thomas' own doctrine of just war is sharply focused on and primarily concerned with the initiation of war (*ius ad bellum*) rather than conduct in war (*ius in bello*) or after war (*ius post bellum*).

It would be a mistake to regard the gaps and silences in Thomas' doctrine of just war as harmless oversights. In particular, his seeming lack of interest in the question of civilian or noncombatant deaths in war is striking. Admittedly, he argues elsewhere that it is sinful to slay the innocent;[17] but it remains unclear whether he considers the guilt or innocence of an individual "enemy" in war to be related to whether he or she is bearing arms. The fact is that Aquinas' understanding of just or legitimate war may be distilled down to several fundamental assertions. Firstly, it is clear that war is the work of laymen and that the relevant laymen may be divided into two categories: sovereigns and soldiers, each with its own appropriate roles and responsibilities. Sovereigns—emperors, kings, princes, governors—alone make the call whether war is rightly warranted and, if so, issue the call to arms, while soldiers—citizens or subjects of the sovereign—must answer the sovereign's call and go to war. It is neither the right nor the responsibility, it would appear, of anyone but the sovereign to weigh the moral merits of a given war. That weighs on the conscience of the "king," while what must concern the soldier is to obey his ruler and, at the same time, to wage war with the right intent and inner disposition—free of hatred, rage, revenge, battle-lust, savagery, or any other dark, corrupting passion or disturbance of soul.

At the sure risk of oversimplification, we might sum up and say that it is left to rulers to declare just wars, and it is up to soldiers to fight clean

16. Ibid. See Augustine, *Contra Faustum*, xxii.74.
17. Thomas Aquinas, *Summa Theologica*, II-II, Qu. 64.

ones. To be sure, Augustine placed far more emphasis on the former than on the latter, perhaps in part because he realized all too well that while sound, ethical judgment might well play a role and even on occasion hold sway before a war begins, the chances that moral reason and virtue might survive and prevail in actual battle were slim indeed. As Thucydides put it so poignantly, "war is a stern teacher,"[18] and its first lesson is just how thin and frail is the veneer that separates civilization from savagery. It is at least fair to say that Aquinas placed greater emphasis on sovereign authority and submission to it than did Augustine. He didn't share his revered predecessor's profound and outspoken suspicion of the public and political order and the coercive powers that went with it. For Augustine, these are a legacy of the fall from grace, a concession foreseen and foreordained by God to lessen the burden of earthly life in a sinful, corrupt world. It is only in such a world that we are better off with political dominion than without it. As R. A. Markus puts it,

> coercive power is part of the essence of political authority. Without it the state is not a state. . . . Political authority, coercive power and its apparatus are what transform society into a state. Society, so we may summarize Augustine's view, has its origins in the order of nature; the state is a dispensation rooted in sin.[19]

Aquinas, on the other hand, an avid student of Aristotle, saw matters altogether differently. Like his distant philosophical mentor, he regarded human beings as political by nature, as God created them to be in the Beginning, before the Fall. While for Augustine there can be nothing "natural" about one man's being subject to another, Aquinas argued that at least one form of dominion, that of free men governed for the sake of the common good, was indeed grounded in nature. This meant that he accorded to the state and its sovereign a fundamental legitimacy and an ethical benefit of the doubt that Augustine was unwilling to grant to the City of Man and its institutions. This fact is a fateful one for the future of just war theory, particularly as embraced and implemented by the Catholic Church. This becomes clear when we consider that to this day the Roman Catholic Church, as well as almost every mainline Christian denomination and sect, fails to outspokenly endorse and publically defend selective conscientious objection to war, much less pacifism. Pope Pius XII, in an address on Christmas

---

18. Thucydides, *Peloponnesian War*, 3.82.

19. Markus, "Two Conceptions," 77–78.

Eve (of all days) in 1948, stated that "complete pacifism is indefensible," a position that Jesuit and Oxford moral theologian Henry Davis set forth a bit more vehemently:

> The pacifist, that is, one who will not, under any circumstances, fight for his country in a just war, if legitimately ordered to do so, is an enemy of his country, and of the human race, for his principles would lead him to be passive to the destruction of all ordered society.[20]

In that case, it would follow that the clergy, prohibited by Thomas and the church from fighting in any war, should be judged to be enemies of the state and of humanity, unless of course sending the laity off to do their fighting for them counts as military service.

In practice if not in principle, any war declared by a recognized sovereign authority for what he or she states is a just cause rightly obligates the subjects of that authority to answer the call to war. It is neither the right nor the responsibility of those who go to war in obedience to the state to second-guess, much less contradict, their ruler's determination and assertion of just cause. It is for warriors, rather, to form a right intention and to look to the condition of their individual souls as they go off and wage that war. In other words, just war theory, as Aquinas presents it, is largely irrelevant to combatants, whose obligation is to do what they are ordered to do and to do it with a pure heart, whatever that means in the heat of battle.

Stepping back and out for a moment from the *Summa* of Aquinas, we are left to wonder about his words on war as they touch down in the lives of nations and individuals. How many states or sovereign authorities, we might ask, have ever declared wars that they have not attempted to justify? Enemies in war always see the other side as somehow in the wrong and themselves as in the right. After all, in the deadly contest of war, both sides must field a team, as it were; and in addition to wanting to win, each side is usually, if not always, convinced that they deserve to win. Recalling the focus of this book, we might further ask whether history reveals moral injury to be a common affliction of rulers. How many emperors, kings, princes, presidents, politicians, or, yes, popes, who have put their lips to the horn of war have suffered from, or at least complained of, moral injury from war? Closer to home, in the recent wars of the twentieth and twenty-first centuries, how many American presidents or members of Congress have suffered

20. Davis, *Moral and Pastoral Theology*, 57.

from PTSD or taken their own lives rather than live any longer with the burden of having declared a war and sent other men and women off to fight it? I believe the answer to be none, a small number when we consider that today, in the United States, an average of eighteen veterans commit suicide every day. It is the warriors who are injured in war, in their bodies and in their souls, and their wounds are all but indifferent to whether the war they fought and suffered was just or unjust. Now, as we return to our historical narrative, we may well share some simmering doubt regarding just how much difference the theories of just war laid out by two brilliant and renowned monks—Aquinas and Augustine—have ever made or could ever make in limiting war as we or any of our warlike predecessors have known and practiced it.

So far, within Catholic theory and practice, we have seen the moral and theological status of war and military service change several times since the Sermon on the Mount. Killing—once forbidden under any circumstance— came to be allowed, so long as it was in the service of the state. War—once the lesser of two evils—was for Thomas and the Scholastics the lesser of two goods. Enlistment in the legions—once suspect at best—became praiseworthy and meritorious, a privilege reserved for Christians. Pacifism—once the common conviction of the Christian community—passed to the clergy as a matter of personal immunity. But theirs was an often pugnacious pacifism, calling for the sword without ever wielding it. Christians had, from the beginning, been quietly grateful for the "necessary" wars fought for their safety and benefit by the pagan, idolatrous legions of Rome. Eventually, once the empire was theirs and its legions marched under the standard of the cross, Christians promoted their wars to the moral rank of just and glorious, particularly when fought against barbarians, their natural enemies. Only one more rung remained to be climbed in the rise of war to the pinnacle of Christian service, and the name of that rung was "holy."

Christians had always been familiar, if not fond, of the concept of holy war from their reading of the Hebrew Scriptures, their Old Testament. Moses, Joshua, and David shone in the violent firmament of heroes who fought in wars commanded by God and waged in his name. While the earliest Christians distanced themselves from these stories, later Christians construed and embraced them as an antidote to the pacifism of the gospels. Jesus appeared to want nothing to do with war, but his heavenly father was of the old breed, as it were, a war god if there ever was one. And he was all that the later, ascendant, and sometimes bellicose church needed to legitimize and bless its effort to remake the Christian image of war and military service.

The signature "holy wars" of Christianity were undeniably the Crusades (late eleventh to late thirteenth centuries), which were preached and promoted by popes, beginning with Urban II, who at the Council of Clermont in 1095 called for a campaign against the Muslim infidels wreaking havoc in the east. He told the assembled Franks that while these were his words, the command conveyed in them came from God. This was sovereign authority of the highest order. Among the rewards he and future crusader popes offered their recruits were the remission of sin and eternal salvation, while refusal to answer the call and "take the cross" would mean excommunication and eternal fire. There were, of course, more tangible rewards to be reaped, not only by knights but also by the papacy.

Our purpose here is not to provide an historical account or assessment of the Crusades but merely to point to them collectively as the most notorious instance of holy war in the history of Christianity, as well as the most extreme expression of just war theory gone raving mad. The extent of that madness might be measured in the words of no less than Saint Bernard, founding Abbot of the Cistercian monastery of Clairvaux, one of the most revered and influential monks and churchmen of the Middle Ages. Commissioned by Pope Eugene III to preach the Second Crusade, Bernard in 1146 wrote to "the Lords and very dear Fathers, the Archbishops and Bishops, with the whole clergy and the faithful people of Eastern France and Bavaria,"[21] announcing that "now is the acceptable time, now is the day of salvation." Though they be sinners—"murderers, robbers, adulterers, perjurers, and those guilty of other crimes"—they will put the Lord in their debt by mounting a campaign to save "the very city of the living God" from the "enemies of the Cross." Their final reward from the Lord will be nothing less than "pardon of sins, and everlasting glory."

Bernard's devout advocacy for the ecclesiastically sanctioned violence of his times also found voice in his treatise titled "In Praise of the New Knighthood," a document that he wrote only after having been urged multiple times to do so. The urging came from Hughes de Payns, a French knight who was cofounder and the first Grand Master of the Knights Templar, an order of "otherworldly warriors" committed to martial mastery and monastic austerity. The often savage and corrupt excesses of secular knights were well known and of deep concern to Bernard, who himself came from

21. For full text of letter cited here, see Robinson, *Readings,* I.330–33.

a background of knighthood. He warned of the risks not only to body but also to soul that a secular knight would inevitably face:

> Whenever you march out, O worldly warrior, you have to worry that killing your foe's body may mean killing your soul, or that by him you may be killed, body and soul both.[22]

Bernard was no pacifist, but neither was he blind to the dark realities of war. He maintained that only with a pure heart and the right motive can killing be anything but evil. Even self-defense, much less hatred, greed, pride, or revenge, failed to qualify. Sustained success in battle—killing without being killed—called for exceptional strategy and prowess, while spiritual survival in battle—killing others without killing your own soul— called for an even more exceptional discipline of soul and will. Nullifying a thousand-year-old ban on monks or clergy in combat, the Knights Templar and other orders like them—knights in arms and under religious vows— rose in part out of a growing conviction that just war and sinless killing were beyond the reach of most knights who had far more control over their horses than they did over themselves. To maintain a pure heart, right intention, and selfless resolve—free of anger, glory, greed, and fear—required a new breed of knight, accustomed to ascetic severity and absolute obedience. Holy wars are not for everyone, but rather for, in Bernard's phrase, "the picked troops of God,"[23] who would kill with the love of God in their hearts and die as martyrs.

Bernard himself never visited the Holy Land. "It is evident," wrote Bernard, "that what is needed there are soldiers to fight rather than monks to pray."[24] In the Knights Templar, the Holy Land got both. These "Knights of Christ," as Bernard called them, were engaged in God's ministry, God's avengers, ridding the world of sin and error. Furthermore, he argued, killing an evil man does not make one a man-killer but rather an evil-killer. Like the true Israelites, they "march into battle as men of peace."[25] Fearless, disciplined, and laser-like in focus and resolve, they represent a formidable fighting force, and when the fight is over they retreat to their monastic quarters where

22. Bernard of Clairvaux, *In Praise*, 35.
23. Ibid., 4.
24. Ibid., 29.
25. Ibid., 47.

> They live in cheerful community and sober company, without wives and without children. So that their evangelical perfection will lack nothing, they dwell united in one family with no personal property whatever, careful to keep the unity of the Spirit in the bond of peace. You may say that the whole multitude has but one heart and one soul to the point that no one follows his own will, but seeks instead to follow the commander.[26]

The Knights Templar, who at first were few in number and lived by the borrowed Rule of Saint Augustine, were formally confirmed by the Council of Troyes in 1128 and given their own monastic rule, based on that of the Cistercians. In 1139 the Templars received papal approval and support, when Pope Innocent II granted them virtual autonomy and created a new rank within the order, that of chaplain brothers, with special privileges and powers, such as the hearing of confessions and the forgiving of sins. All of the monks took the vows of poverty, chastity, and obedience and were meant to keep them. How rigorously these vows were originally enforced is suggested by the fact that any monk who kept any money to himself was expelled at once from the order, and any dead monk found with money in his possession could not be buried in consecrated soil, nor were his brother monks expected to pray for his soul. With regard to their vow of chastity, the Templars were forbidden not only sexual relations with women but any intimacy whatsoever with the opposite sex, including the kissing of one's own "mother, sister, aunt or any other."[27] The detailed statutes of their rule[28] numbered nearly seven hundred and addressed every aspect of Templar common life, whether in cloister or combat, stating, for example, that killing a Christian or going over to the Saracens would bring immediate expulsion from the order, while lowering the banner in battle or charging without permission would mean the loss of one's monastic habit or robes. No moment of the day or night, nor aspect of their lives, was left unregulated. It could be suggested that they made today's Marines look like Yippies. In an attempt to sum up the remarkable phenomenon of the warrior-monk, Bernard wrote,

> I don't know if it would be more appropriate to refer to them as monks or as soldiers, or whether it would perhaps be better to

26. Ibid., 45–46.

27. Upton-Ward, *Rule of the Templars*, 36.

28. The Rule of the Knights Templar, beginning with the "Primitive Rule," evolved across 150 years.

recognize them as being both, for they lack neither monastic meekness nor military might. What can we say about this, except that this is the Lord's doing, and it is marvelous in our eyes.[29]

The repute of the Templars, however, unraveled eventually, as the wealth and power of the order became objects of suspicion and envy. Accusations of idolatry, heresy, and immorality abounded, and the Inquisition descended on the order, extracting confessions of heresy from some of its members under torture. Pope Clement V dissolved the Templars in 1312, and two years later the order's last Grand Master was burned at the stake. It is doubtful whether Bernard of Clairvaux, long since dead, would have regarded this too as "the Lord's doing."

The church's experiment with warrior-monks is of particular interest to the concerns of this book because it suggests that Christians were all too aware that even in the most just of all wars, holy wars declared by the highest authority on earth, killing—the killing of infidels, no less—could be and in many cases was sinful, not for lack of just cause but for lack of right intention. And "right intention," the church had always known, was as difficult to sustain in battle as it was in bed. Since the time of Antony and the Desert Monks of the late third and fourth centuries, monks (or at least some monks) had the reputation of being able to lie next to a naked woman without distraction, much less desire. This, it would seem, was precisely the kind and level of control required of a warrior to kill without animus or fear and to conquer without pride, revenge, or avarice. Although the church never said so, the warriors it truly needed to fight its wars would have been best described as angels—the sword-wielding sort—like the heavenly legions led by Archangel Michael. This was exactly how the holy ascetics of Egypt and Syria had once been regarded, minus the swords. In the Middle Ages, the Templars and other warrior-monks like them were as close as the church came to enlisting angels to fight for the Lord.

The truth is that men can never be angels and, if they could, we may wonder whether they would ever find the wars they were being asked to fight to be just. With a dearth of angels at hand, the task is left to men, and men all too often go dark in war—dark in death or dark in life, or both. And they can't help it. Just or unjust, war leaves scars, on souls as well as bodies. "For there are many things," wrote Pope Gregory the Great to Augustine of Canterbury, "which are lawful and permitted, and yet we are somewhat

---

29. Bernard of Clairvaux, *In Praise*, 48.

defiled in doing them."[30] This recognition, as well as "the continuance of the age-old view . . . that engaging in warfare even at the command of the prince and in a just cause involves grave sin,"[31] found expression in the numerous *Libri Poenitentiales* or "Penitentials" in wide use for several centuries in the British Isles and across the continent. The first of these books appeared in Britain and Ireland in the early sixth century. Not unlike mandatory sentencing guidelines today, their purpose was to provide appropriate and uniform penances for various sins. In the sacrament of confession, the absolution of sin requires the priest-confessor to impose and the confessing sinner to perform a penance suited to each infraction. As a rule, the early Irish and British penitentials, as well as those that emerged in the ensuing four centuries across Europe, imposed penances for killing in war comparable to those prescribed by such church fathers as Cyprian, Basil, and Isidore, as well as by the fourth-century church councils of Arles and Nicaea. Commonly this meant a straightforward forty-day penance, but some penitentials, such as the Arundel Penitential, dating from the late tenth century, were appreciably more harsh and detailed in their recommendations:

> In the first place, anyone who kills an enemy while trying to repulse an invasion of his own country is required to do three years' penance. A distinction is then drawn between royal battles and those waged only by princes. Killing of a man in a royal battle, it is said, always brings a one-year penance. If a public war is being waged by a prince, however, a further distinction must be made between just and unjust wars. If there is any doubt about whether the war is just or unjust, a penance of two years is to be imposed upon anyone involved in a homicide. Even if the war is thought to be just, those who kill during the course of the battle are still to do penance for one year.[32]

Surely, one of the most illuminating medieval documents regarding the imposition of penances for killing in war is the Penitential Ordinance of 1067, issued in the year following the Battle of Hastings. Among the detailed and severe penances imposed by the ordinance on the Norman knights who fought with William the Conqueror on Senlac Hill are the following:

---

30. Bede, *Ecclesiastical History*, I.27.
31. Cowdrey, "Bishop Ermenfrid," 237–38.
32. Cited in Verkamp, *Moral Treatment*, 5.

Anyone who knows that he killed a man in the great battle must do penance for one year for each man that he killed.

Anyone who wounded a man, and does not know whether he killed him or not, must do penance for forty days for each man he thus struck (if he can remember the number), either continuously or at intervals.

Anyone who does not know the number of those he wounded or killed must, at the discretion of his bishop, do penance for one day in each week for the remainder of his life; or, if he can, let him redeem his sin by a perpetual alms, either by building or by endowing a church.

The clerks who fought, or who were armed for fighting, must do penance as if they had committed these sins in their own country, for they are forbidden by the canons to do battle.

Those who fought merely for gain are to know that they owe penance as for a homicide.

Those who fought as in a public war have been allotted a penance of three years by their bishops out of mercy.

The archers who killed some and wounded others, but are necessarily ignorant as to how many, must do penance as for three Lents.[33]

It goes without saying that the imposition of penances for killing in war—a practice that dated from the early centuries of Christianity and continued into the eleventh century—was difficult to reconcile with the waging of holy war. Military service in holy wars, after all, was held to be both compulsory and meritorious. The Crusades of the High Middle Ages that defined the genre were mostly declared and recruited by the currently reigning pope. Those who failed to answer his call and take up the crusader's cross were often threatened with excommunication and the damnation of their souls, while those who took up arms and the cross were promised anything from the remission of their sins to a guarantee of eternal salvation. However incongruous it was to impose penances on crusaders for killing God's enemies in God's wars, this practice survived to the end of the eleventh century. One of the additional anomalies of the period during which the crusaders were simultaneously serving God and staining their hands and souls, was that a common reward for military service came in the form of papal indulgences that annulled the penances imposed for that same service.

33. Ibid., 6.

There is no consensus among historians regarding why the Christian practice of imposing penances on returning warriors for their wartime killing became outmoded and fell into disuse. It may be that the theology of holy war and the experience of the Crusades made the practice untenable. Curiously and perhaps tellingly, Thomas Aquinas had nothing much to say on the matter of the Crusades and holy war; and, with the Thomistic doctrine of just war in place, the church had little to say that was helpful to those who returned from a sanctioned war in moral pain. The spiritual distress and desolation of returning warriors was from now on their secret, their private problem, as it were, incomprehensible to others, a phantom pain felt in a missing or invisible extremity. It was not, could not be, "real" nor have any relevance in the real world. In the ensuing centuries, the definition and adjudication of just war would be increasingly left not to theologians but to lawyers. It was a matter to be settled between sovereigns and states, a matter of international not ecclesiastical law. It was out of the hands of soldiers. That is, until it came to the fighting and the killing and the dying and the coming home in confusion.

7

Early Modern Europe

Warriors and Lawyers

O PENING THE GATES OF war was relatively easy. Closing them again, even partway, was to prove more difficult. In the history of Christian Europe, the first was the work of moralists and theologians and the second was a task eventually left to lawyers. It should not come to anyone's surprise that the dogs of war, once loosed, did not and do not take readily to the leash.

As we have already seen, for Augustine and later for Aquinas—the two founding fathers of the just war doctrine—the question at hand was simple and straightforward: Is war so essentially evil that a Christian cannot go there without grave sin? The specific sin that most concerned them was the violation of love, the love of God and neighbor. In his *Summa Theologica*, Thomas Aquinas situated his brief treatise on war broadly within his discussion of the three theological virtues of faith, hope, and love, and more specifically in that part focused on love and the vices or evils opposed to it. "If I have all faith, so as to remove mountains," sang Paul in his hymn to love penned to the Corinthians, "but do not have love, I am nothing. . . . And now faith, hope, and love abide, these three; and the greatest of these is love" (1 Cor 13:2, 13). To sin against love is no light matter, and if war is such a sin, then it cannot be condoned.

The would-be solution that Augustine found and that Aquinas confirmed to permit war and to preserve love was to wage the former with the latter, to love and do what must be done. The tough paternal love of God the Father and of the heads of every Christian household—punitive, corrective, and caring—provided the needed paradigm for a Christian love that could be carried into battle rather than trampled underfoot there.

Both Augustine and Aquinas focused on the just initiation of war—*ius ad bellum*—the just or virtuous way of *going to war*, and agreed on its ingredients: sovereign authority (*auctoritas principis*), just cause (*iusta causa*), and right intention (*recta intentio*).[1] Like the three designated settings of a combination lock, they served to open the way to war without sin, war without guilt, even war with merit. In all fairness, there is ample evidence in their writings that both Augustine and Aquinas shared a moral presumption against war and killing and saw these as a last and unfortunate resort. Regrettably, such a presumption was not their legacy. Their prescription for just war was a formula for enablement, not deterrence. Each element, however, begged for clarification. Who qualified as a sovereign authority? Who was to say whether a cause was just? And how could anyone judge my or anyone else's intentions when they reside—or should we say hide—so far beyond public scrutiny that they are truly for "me to know and for you (unless you are God) to find out."

Of equal or greater concern was that the just war doctrine sketched by Augustine and Aquinas left the warrior on the brink of battle, where war begins but not where it ends. They offered little or no guidance regarding what was acceptable and unacceptable in the conduct of war (*ius in bello*) and after the war was won, or lost (*ius post bellum*). Perhaps they suspected that as soon as a war is underway ethical considerations regarding *modus debitus* (proportional means or right conduct) are as unlikely to survive as are the crops or wildflowers under an army's feet. Once armed, angry, and authorized, boys will be boys. But surely there must be limits. Indeed, a forest of moral issues and questions awaited warriors, then as now, so soon as the battle is joined: whether noncombatants—those whose only crime was to be in the wrong place at the wrong time or on the "other side" of the conflict—could be freely killed and their possessions seized; whether enemy combatants who wish to surrender or have already surrendered may be summarily executed; whether a defeated foe merits a measure of respect or mere annihilation; whether the lands and possessions of a defeated people

---

1. Francisco Suarez, a Jesuit, who wrote in the sixteenth and seventeenth centuries on the ethics of war and peace in the tradition of Aquinas and Vitoria, replaced *recta intentio* with *modus debitus* or "right conduct"—*ad bellum, in bello,* and *post bellum.*

belong to the victor in a spirit of "winner take all." These were but a few of the countless moral and legal queries raised but not yet resolved by the just war theory of Augustine, adopted by Aquinas, and in good time endorsed by the church.

The pivotal fact here is that the just war doctrine first proposed by Augustine was a theological theory, and like any theory it required to be tested. Theories—in theology no less than in physics—are not made true by virtue of their being asserted. Even general acceptance is no measure of their validity. They must survive the test of time, experience, and change. As it happens, the medieval Christian theory of just war, as we shall see, did not in the end survive these tests, which is not to say that it was altogether abandoned. Disproven theories don't automatically die. Often they take on new lives. So it is with the just war theory. But in saying this we are far ahead of ourselves. What we must trace here, in an inevitably cursory manner, is the development and testing of that theory across the contentious and turbulent span from the early codification of ecclesiastical or canon law in the twelfth century to the birth of international law in the seventeenth century.

Augustine and Aquinas were moralists and theologians, not lawyers. As such, they were concerned with the prescriptions of divine law, with virtue and sin, rather than with positive or conventional law. Ecclesiastical or canon law lay somewhere between these two. The Roman Catholic Church—a worldly polity with otherworldly titles and claims—structured itself in many ways after the Roman Empire whose institutional genome it had in part inherited. Part of this inheritance was its legal system, complete with law codes, courts, lawyers, and judges. We will focus here on its law codes, whose principal sources were predictably diverse: the Bible, the writings of the church fathers, the canons or decrees of church councils and synods, papal declarations and letters, episcopal statutes, collections of ancient Roman law (particularly the Code of the Emperor Justinian), and eventually natural law, with the rediscovery of the works of Aristotle in the twelfth and thirteenth centuries. Needless to say, not all of these disparate voices were on the same page regarding the ethics and rules of war.

A decisive moment in the collection and codification of canon law came with the monumental work of Gratian, a Camaldolese monk, scholar, and jurist, who at Bologna around 1140 completed his *Concordia discordantium canonum*, simply and more often referred to as Gratian's *Decretum*. This vast assembly and orchestration of close to four thousand texts, arguments, counterarguments, opinions, authorities, and carefully crafted case studies was soon adopted as the definitive text for the study of canon law at the most prestigious nascent law schools of the Latin West—Bologna, Orleans, and Cologne. Succeeding generations of European legal scholars studied, commented on, debated, and annotated the *Decretum*, thus confirming its foundational place and importance in the centuries-long gestation and development of ecclesiastical law.

Of central interest to our discussion here, of course, are Gratian's assertions and arguments regarding those laws governing Christian warfare. Among his many aims and endeavors in the *Decretum*, Gratian took it upon himself to construct a thorough and concise theological justification for Christian engagement in war. And "Christian engagement," of course, meant the church's engagement. Gratian sought to leave no doubt in anyone's mind that the church's temporal authority, like that of the state, included the right to wage war, arguing that any war undertaken with divine authorization does not violate the fifth commandment, prohibiting the taking of human life. Crucial for this and countless other arguments and assertions was his conflation of divine authority and ecclesiastical authority. While he was at it, Gratian also provided what he and the majority of his successors considered to be a cogent case for the legitimate and moral right of both church and state to impose appropriate correction and punishment on heretics and miscreants, including torture and execution. An addendum here was his claim that heretics have no right whatsoever to own personal property and may be righteously dispossessed of all such. The writings of Augustine and the "authority" that had accrued to them were especially helpful to him in making these arguments, but Gratian drew upon countless disparate sources—sacred and secular—in his determinations. Conspicuously absent in his treatment of warfare and penal violence were the teachings of Jesus in the gospels.

This avoidance of the gospels in the church's justification of war and sanctioning of state and ecclesiastical violence marked nearly all of the theological, moral, and legal texts produced within the just war tradition, whose authors rarely made any reference or appeal to the words and example of Jesus, unless to neuter them with the subtle knife of allegory. Consequently, with the gospels extracted and neutralized, there was not enough left in the Bible to make the case against war. Next to the gospel narratives, the longest single narrative in the Bible focused on David, to whom defenders of Christian violence often turned for inspiration and support. In the conveniently refracted light of a distorted faith, David served as a paradigm for divinely ordained warrior-kings, or popes, despite the fact that, under a more forensic light, he might be indicted as a serial killer. Indeed, several centuries after Gratian, long after the die had been cast, one of the most revered churchmen and scholars of Christendom, Erasmus of Rotterdam, the "Tutor of Europe," made much the same point with a poignancy and eloquence that was nevertheless largely ignored:

> It can be argued that papal laws do not condemn all war. Augustine too approves it somewhere. Again, St. Bernard praises some soldiers. True enough, but Christ himself, and Peter, and Paul, always teach the opposite. Why does their authority carry less weight than that of Augustine or Bernard? Augustine does not disapprove of war in one or two passages, but the whole philosophy of Christ argues against war. Nowhere do the Apostles approve it, and as for those holy doctors who are alleged to have approved of war in one or two passages, how many passages are there where they condemn and curse it? Why do we gloss over all these and seize on the bits which support our wickedness? In fact, anyone who examines the matter more closely will find that none of them approves of the kind of war which is usually fought today.[2]

We would be mistaken, however, if we were to imagine that the church and its people were won over to the justification of Christian warfare as soon as Augustine made his case. In fact, it required centuries for the church to reach anything like a quorum, much less a consensus, in war's favor. Indeed, the church was deeply divided over the legitimacy of war for centuries. Notable canonists, ranking members of the papal court, and countless others among the clergy and laity agreed with Peter Damian— a Benedictine monk, a cardinal in the court of Pope Gregory VII, and a Doctor of the church—when in the eleventh century he argued that "in no circumstances is it licit to take up arms in defense of the faith of the universal church; still less should men rage in battle for its earthly and transitory goods."[3] The truth was that, despite the frequent endorsement of the just war doctrine of Augustine,

> right into the second half of the eleventh century, and therefore on the very eve of the First Crusade, the Christian West was also teaching that killing or wounding in warfare, however legitimate

2. Erasmus, *Collected Works*, 27:104.
3. *Ep.* 4.9 (PL 144:316), cited in Cowdrey, "Genesis of the Crusades," 19.

the cause, was gravely sinful and merited severe penance. From this point of view, warfare was far from having the Church's blessing and approval: it stood under its condemnation. Far from being a legitimate service in the name of Christ, the profession of arms was not really fitting for a Christian man.[4]

The church was clearly or, to be more honest, confusedly, of two minds on the question of Christian participation in war until the late twelfth century. For centuries it had been blessing the banners that knights carried into battle, and at least by the tenth century it had developed formulas for the blessing of swords and other weapons, as well as a liturgical ritual for the investiture and dubbing of knights. The following *Oratio super militantes* or prayer for men going into battle has survived from the same period:

> Bless, O Lord, your servants who bend their heads before you. Pour on them your stablishing grace. In the warfare in which they are to be tested, preserve them in health and good fortune. Wherever and whyever they ask for your help, be speedily present to protect and defend them.[5]

So which was it to be? Was "the profession of arms . . . not really fitting for a Christian man," or were men-at-arms "servants" of the Lord? More than any one man, Pope Gregory VII resolved the church's deep dissonance over the moral legitimacy of warfare. So far from its being essentially evil, Gregory proclaimed it to be at times both necessary and fully acceptable, even honorable and potentially meritorious. Gregory was, as it happened, only the first of a number of what might be called "war popes," who saw knighthood and the profession of arms as a worthy Christian vocation in the service of the church and its interests. From this point on, the just war theory in its broadest formulation was a matter of Christian doctrine. While centuries of Christian theologians, canonists, and legists debated its details, true dissidents were few and ineffectual. Christian pacifism was essentially a dead letter and the New Testament, on issues of war and punitive violence, a censored text. When it came to war, the church was, it seems, irreversibly complicit and compromised.

> In the medieval theories aggressive war and non-combatant immunity received little attention. Fighting and dying in warfare was a function of the knightly class. When their cause was just, there

4. Cowdrey, "Genesis of the Crusades," 17.
5. Cited in ibid., 16.

were only vague moral limits on their conduct, such as condemnation of the lust for conquest. Rather than attempting to eliminate war altogether, the scholastics more realistically and modestly tried to reduce the incidence of violence, but even here their effectiveness was limited by their feudal bias.[6]

Having permitted war, the medieval church was nevertheless concerned with, and at times committed to, limiting its reach and savagery. The just war theory that the church—pope, clergy, theologians, and princes—accepted was a theory of limited, not total, war. When the church of the first few centuries prayed for the success of the pagan emperor and his legions, they were concerned with their safety and security, with preserving the Pax Romana that allowed the church to grow and flourish. So too, now in a Christian empire, Augustine, in proposing a formula for just war, was concerned with securing the state and the church from its enemies, within and without—barbarians, heretics, and schismatics. The just war theory, put simply, had its origin in fear—the fear of chaos—and the corresponding longing for security and order.

It is likely that no one, however, least of all Augustine, foresaw the level and kind of chaos that rocked Christian Europe a thousand years after the birth of Christ and as soon as warfare, in theory, won the official, if conditional, blessing of the church. Europe was literally coming apart now, as the *respublica Christiana* unraveled and disintegrated into a patchwork of competing sovereign states—national monarchies, principalities, city-states, duchies, baronies, and a diminished Holy Roman Empire that had already begun its slow but sure dinosauric march into obsolescence and extinction. Post-Carolingian France devolved into the "wild west" of Europe, and most of Spain—fallen to infidel invaders—now comprised the Caliphate of Cordoba. Nothing short of anarchy prevailed as knights, barons, and robber bands had their way. Warfare was taken up as a favored pastime by the upper classes, kings and knights who apparently had nothing better to do than to wreak havoc on the helpless. If this was not the "war of all against all" later declared by Thomas Hobbes to be the natural and original condition of our species, it was close. Churches, monasteries, convents, pilgrims, merchants, farmers—anyone or anywhere without armor or arms—fell prey to the caprice of random, unprovoked violence, and ordinary people who wanted nothing more than to carry on with their lives in peace looked to princes and knights for protection.

6. Russell, *Just War*, 308.

The church, in embracing the just war theory, had anticipated and conditionally legitimized three types of wars: wars declared by God, wars declared by the church, and wars declared by a sovereign authority. But much if not most of the violence that now infected Europe like a plague represented none of these. Canonists and theologians distinguished between public wars, corresponding to the three genres of just war cited above, and private wars, which could only rarely be judged just. Private wars were, for the most part, blatant brigandage blown large, whose only aims were revenge, plunder, or the perverse thrill of slaughter and destruction. On this form of war the church was of one mind, condemning it as gravely sinful. However much the church was willing to concede that at least some public wars violated neither the fifth commandment nor Christian charity, private wars fell beyond the pale of ecclesiastical permissiveness.

What was worst about the wars that first ravaged early medieval Europe was the fact that in them Christians were killing their fellow Christians. Wholesale Christian-on-Christian violence was on a very fundamental level inconceivable and certainly irreconcilable with the core of Christian faith. It cut the church to the quick. Here it was impossible to silence the commandment of love, the last will and testament, as it were, of Christ:

> I give you a new commandment, that you love one another. Just as I have loved you, you also should love one another. By this everyone will know that you are my disciples, if you have love for one another. (John 13:34–35)

Yet even when confronted with so grave a scandal and horror as inter-Christian violence, the church was officially unwilling to condemn all warfare and actually unable to call a simple halt to its most outrageous forms. Instead, the church set about trying to establish and enforce some tolerable limits. One such effort became known as the Peace of God. This movement first emerged in southern and southwestern France and sought to immunize the church's own—its monasteries, convents, churches, and property as well as clergy, religious, and pilgrims—from attack and injury. Soon its protective arm was extended further to protect townspeople, merchants, and peasants, together with their homes, lands, and possessions. The Peace of God as proclaimed in an assembly convened by Archbishop Gumbald of Aquitania secunda (the Province of Bordeaux) in 989 made clear the ultimate ecclesiastical sanction facing anyone who violated its provisions:

1. Anathema for violators of churches: if anyone breaks into a sacred church, or violently removes anything thence, unless he makes satisfaction, let him be anathema.

2. Anathema for spoilers of the poor: if anyone robs peasants or other poor of a sheep, ox, ass, cow, goat, or pigs, unless by the other's fault, and if he neglect to make full reparation, let him be anathema.

3. Anathema for those who assault the clergy: if anyone attacks, captures or assaults a priest or deacon or any clergyman, who is not carrying arms (that is, shield, sword, coat of mail and helmet), but quietly going on his way or remaining at home, that sacrilegious man shall be held to be cast forth from the holy church of God, unless he makes satisfaction, after the clergyman has been examined by his bishop to see if he was at fault.[7]

Originally, as is clear from the above, the church enforced the Peace of God with its threat of excommunication. Soon, however, as the Peace of God spread across Europe,[8] it won the support of many kings and princes who attached more tangible forms of punishment to its infractions. In addition to providing some real respite from the senseless violence of the times, the Peace of God inspired and lent support to the idea and eventual inclusion of noncombatant immunity amongst the provisions of just war legislation. In addition, the Peace of God movement soon spawned a second and similar campaign to limit medieval warfare. This was known as the Truce of God, and its purpose was to confine warfare to certain days of the week and certain times of the year. Admittedly, in a simple count of days allotted to either peace or war, war won the lion's share; yet it was significant that the

7. Laffan, *Select Documents*, 19.

8. It is worthy of note that three hundred years before the assembly at Charroux, the Irish Church, together with "the men of Ireland and Britain," enacted a document known to us as the *Cáin Adamnáin* or the "Law of Adamnan" at the Synod of Birr in 696–97. Adamnan was abbot of Iona and the biographer of Columba, one of the three pillars (together with Patrick and Bridgit) of early Irish Christianity. Adamnan sought to shield, in particular, clerics, women, and children, as well as their households and holdings, from the endemic violence of the Irish tribal system of the day. Remarkably for the times, the Law of Adamnan prescribed severe penalties not only for rape but also for domestic violence and any unwanted sexual advances on a woman, such as "putting a hand in her girdle . . . [or a] tearing of her dress . . . [or] making a gentlewoman blush by imputing unchastity to her" (Meyer, *Cáin Adamnáin*, 50–51). This may well represent the first law in the West, if not in the world, that formally prohibits and assigns meaningful penalties not only for domestic and sexual abuse but for what we today label sexual harassment.

church was able to spare its most hallowed days and seasons from the chaos and pollution of organized slaughter.

The earliest Truce of God was proclaimed in 1027 in the diocese of Elne, situated in the heart of the eastern Pyrenees. This was followed twenty-seven years later by a more extensive and influential proclamation of both the Peace and the Truce of God at the Council of Narbonne, whose provisions included the following:

> 1. First, we order that no Christian slay his fellow Christian. For he who kills a Christian, without doubt sheds the blood of Christ. If anyone unjustly kills a man, he shall pay the penalty according to the law.
>
> 2. We confirm the truce of God, which was long ago established by us and now is broken by evil men. Henceforth it shall be faithfully observed by all. Accordingly we adjure in God's name every Christian not to do hurt to any other Christian from sunset on Wednesday till sunrise on Monday.
>
> 3. From the first Sunday in Advent till the octave of Epiphany; from the Sunday before Lent till the octave of Easter; from the Sunday before Ascension Day till the octave of Whitsunday; and on the following feasts and their vigils—those of St. Mary, St. John Baptist, apostles, St. Peter in Chains, Justus and Pastor, St. Laurence, St. Michael, All Saints, St. Martin; and in the four periods of Ember Days: we forbid any Christian to attack another Christian during any of the said fasts, feasts and vigils or to insult him or to seize his property. . . .
>
> 9. Olive trees, which, we read, were used as a sign that peace had returned to the earth at the time of the flood, and from whose oil the holy chrism is made shall be so strictly protected that no Christian shall dare to cut them down or injure them or seize their fruit.
>
> 10. Sheep and their pastors, while tending them, shall also be under the truce of God on all days in all places.[9]

In the next century, the Lateran Council of 1339, the second general council of the Western church, confirmed the core elements of the Peace and Truce of God and added some related sanctions of its own, condemning lethal jousts and tournaments, denying Christian burial to anyone killed in knightly blood sports, and excommunicating incendiaries and any missile

---

9. Laffan, *Selected Documents*, 20–21.

troops who would employ the "deadly and God-detested art of stingers and archers . . . against Christians and Catholics."[10]

Apart from the fact that the Peace of God and Truce of God lost momentum and proved in the end to have little lasting effect, we may well be troubled by their outspoken focus on violence visited on "Christians and Catholics." Without diminishing the scandal of internecine Christian warfare or denying the theological claim that "he who kills a Christian, without doubt sheds the blood of Christ," we might wonder to what extent the church was concerned about he who kills a non-Christian. At the same time as the church endeavored to hold its members to a higher standard of morality, that same standard was unashamedly biased and exclusive. Regarding war and much else, the church brandished two sets of rules, one for Christians and another for everyone else. This may have seemed only common sense at the time, but in retrospect it falls a good deal short of common decency.

In addition to the Peace and Truce of God, the church employed another decidedly bellicose solution to the deadly chaos in Europe. This was to recruit and redirect its knights and their seemingly unquenchable aggression in directions that served rather than savaged the church's designs and interests. And these new endeavors would not, in theory, call for Christians to kill other Christians. The church, for instance, encouraged Christian knights to undertake the reconquest of Granada, but the liberation of Spain from Muslim rule was not finally accomplished until several centuries later, in 1492. Another failed effort to foster peace while making religious war abroad came in 1074, when Pope Gregory VII proposed to lead an armed expedition to the east to lend martial assistance to Byzantine Christians in their struggle against the Turks. But Gregory's premature and ill-conceived scheme to enlist and unite the knights of Europe in his *militia Christi*—a military attack force at papal beck and call—found few takers and fell quite flat. It was Pope Urban II, who at Clermont in 1095 seized the right moment and found the right words to launch the First Crusade. And so an age of ideological or "holy" war was launched. Most of the wars witnessed and either condoned or condemned by the church up to this point had been fought over interests, rights, or personal feuds. The Crusades were different. They marked the beginning of Christian total war, wars of annihilation—God's wars, willed by God, fought for God's causes by God's armies. In these wars Christian warriors were permitted, even encouraged,

10. Schroeder, *Disciplinary Decrees*, 213.

to "take the gloves off," as it were, inasmuch as they were pitted against the enemies of God or at least of the church. Few saw a distinction here worthy of notice.

Once again, as in the earliest days of the Christian church, war—further from home in every sense—became easier to justify. Wars against "barbarians" had from the beginning of Christian history presented less of a challenge to the church's conscience than wars in which Christian blood was shed on both sides. The question that hung in the air was what the church and her knights would do when there were no more barbarians. This dilemma was postponed, however, by the discovery of the New World and the age of overseas conquests that soon followed. The conquest of the Americas raised a new and unique challenge to Christian just war theory, a challenge that the famed Spanish moral theologian Franciscus de Victoria undertook to meet. Victoria breathed new life into scholastic theology and brought to it his own remarkably broad and rich command of sacred and secular learning. A luminary of the University of Salamanca, Victoria was often consulted on matters of conscience by the Holy Roman Emperor and by other rulers of the day, and is to this day regarded as one of the earliest pioneers and founders of international law. As such, he is best known for two lectures he delivered in 1539—*De Indis* ("On the Amerindians") and *De Iure Belli* ("On the Law of War"). The surviving texts of these lectures, first published in 1557, were not from his hand, but were instead composed after his death from the notes of his "auditors," who in this case comprised virtually the entire university community gathered to hear his annual *relectiones*. These two writings—*De Indis* and its sequel, *De Iure Belli*—were in fact the first developed works of any notable Christian philosopher solely focused on the subject of war. And none too soon.

The conquest and colonization of the New World by Christian Spain raised a plethora of issues and questions simply not addressed in existing canon or civil law. In the absence of established law, the Spanish crown and its conquistadors were making up their rules as they went, while at the same time Victoria, for his part, undertook to examine the titles or claims advanced by the Spanish to justify their systematic and determined domination of the New World. For starters, Victoria pointed out that Christopher Columbus first set out with only one such "title" in his pocket—the "right of discovery," which comes down to "finders keepers." Victoria, however, pointed out that this right properly belongs only to those who discover uninhabited territory, making them its first occupants. This, however, was not what Columbus had found in the New World. Instead, he had come upon a land that was "new" to him but not to those who already happily inhabited it in peace.

Clearly the deck was stacked against the first nations of the Americas, and not only by the disproportionate brute force that the Spanish applied to the task of conquest; they seemed to have God, the church, and all that was right and just against them. The pope and the emperor, each for his own part, claimed rightful sovereign authority over the entire earth. And, as for the "savage" aborigines of the Americas, it was claimed that they had no rights of ownership or sovereignty at all, due to their pagan unbelief, idolatry, unsound minds, and sinful lives. Canon and civil law in Christian Europe offered some real protection of the rights and claims of Christians, but the "exotics" of the Americas fell outside such protections. They were little more than prey.

In Victoria's response to these and other titles or claims asserted by the conquerors and their enablers, Victoria denied and dismantled, one at a time, every justification proffered by those in power to defend what they were clearly willing and determined to do in any event. In order to accomplish this, he argued that the ethical and theological issues at hand were not in this instance within the proper purview of canon or conventional law, but were instead matters of conscience to be decided by divine rather than human law. By divine law he did not mean those precepts and counsels revealed in Scripture, much less the codes of canon law, but rather the "law of creation" or "natural law" to which all human beings have equal access and appeal. It is, in the words of Thomas Aquinas, "nothing else than the rational creature's participation in eternal law."[11] It is called "natural" because its prescriptions are inscribed in our very nature, and so it represents the universal and immutable foundation of all human law. Christian law may enhance and perfect natural law but may never contradict it; for to contradict it would be to quarrel with God the Creator of all things. It was Thomas Aquinas who first and fully welcomed the return of Greek philosophy, most notably that of Aristotle, to the West and allowed it to infuse his theological writings with pre-Christian rational thought, of which natural law was an honored offspring. Franciscus de Victoria, for his part, was a committed, though not altogether uncritical, Thomist, and so, armed with the natural law tradition, he took on the Christian casuistry of those who would dispossess and destroy entire civilizations in what they claimed to be just

11. Thomas Aquinas, *Summa Theologica*, I-II, Qu. 94.

wars. What allowed him to do so was his conviction and claim that, while the Amerindians did not share a common faith, history, or culture with their counterparts in Christian Europe, they did share a common humanity with them, and by virtue of this shared humanity they were decidedly equal participants in the *ius gentium*, the law of nations.

We can do no more here than indicate the core conclusions of Victoria's case against the claims of Spain to be waging legitimate and just wars of conquest in the New World. Arguing that "the Emperor is not the lord of the whole earth,"[12] and similarly that "the Pope has not the whole earth for his sphere,"[13] he concluded that they have simply no temporal or spiritual jurisdiction over the native peoples of the Americas. Regarding the claim that the nonbelievers and especially those who refuse to believe in Christianity after it has been preached to them have no rights before the law, Victoria argued that "this is not a reason which justifies making war on them and depriving them of their property,"[14] and further that "Christian princes can not, even by the authorization of the Pope, restrain the Indians from sins against the law of nature or punish them because of those sins."[15] To sum up, when the Spanish "discovered" them,

> the aborigines undoubtedly had true dominion in both public and private matters, just like Christians, and . . . neither their princes nor private persons could be despoiled of their property on the ground of their not being true owners. . . . The people in question were in peaceable possession of their goods, both publicly and privately. Therefore, unless the contrary is shown, they must be treated as owners and not be disturbed in their possession unless cause be shown.[16]

Regarding "cause," Victoria, in *De Iure Belli*, stated quite clearly that "there is a single and only just cause for commencing a war, namely, a wrong received."[17] And the Spanish, up to this time, had received no such wrong. It is a tragedy on several levels, however, that Victoria did not leave it at this. Instead, perhaps in the name of intellectual thoroughness, he offered and briefly considered over a dozen additional titles or claims that might

12. Victoria, *De Indis*, II.1.

13. Ibid., II.3.

14. Ibid., II.15.

15. Ibid., II.16.

16. Ibid., I.24, 3

17. Victoria, *De Iure Belli*, 13.

be alleged to justify Spanish conquest and possession of the Americas, half of which he regarded as inadequate and seven or eight of which he judged to be just and legitimate. The latter include violations of what he held to be international law or natural law or both, such as the denial of hospitality to well-intentioned visitors from abroad, the refusal to allow trade with foreigners, any prohibition against preaching the Christian faith, or any persecution of Christian converts. Needless to say, after having been invaded and slaughtered by the Spanish, there were those among the Amerindians who were less than hospitable to the Spanish and less than eager to trade with them, much less allow them to preach a religion that could rightly have been seen as complicit with their conquest, dispossession, and in some cases enslavement. And so Franciscus de Victoria, who had been such a formidable voice against the Spanish *conquista,* in the end provided grounds for its acceptance.

Before we leave the work of Victoria, there are two questions of pivotal significance for the future of just war theory that he raised and addressed in *De Iure Belli* and that we would do well to discuss briefly at this point. The first of these asks whether it is conceivable in war that both sides might have a just cause. The possibility of "two just causes" or "simultaneous justice" in war was a point of ongoing debate among medieval and early modern moralists and jurists and was obviously not a slight matter. We may wonder whether such a hypothetical war would be especially just or doubly unjust? And just how hypothetical is it anyway? After all, as Erasmus later put it,

> Who is there who does not think his cause just? Amid so many shifts and changes in human affairs, amid the making and breaking of many agreements and treaties, how could anyone not find a pretext, if any sort of pretext is enough to start a war?[18]

Of course, thinking one's cause is just is not the same as having a truly just cause. Victoria, while he asserts unequivocally that there can be no war in which both sides have just cause, also admits that in war it is often the case that both sides truly think their cause to be just. In such instances, one side, according to Victoria, is in ignorance of the truth. Here he distinguishes between "vincible ignorance" and "invincible ignorance" (a term borrowed from his mentor Aquinas). The former is when the mistaken party should know better and consequently should be held responsible for its blindness.

18. Erasmus, *Collected Works,* 27:104.

An example of culpable or vincible ignorance would be that of a deliberately careless or self-deceived sovereign who rushes into war without serious scrutiny of his own cause. "Invincible ignorance," on the other hand, is no one's fault and describes those instances when a sovereign has exercised all due diligence and in perfectly good faith wages what he mistakenly thinks is a just war.

The poignant and unavoidable reality here is that in practice each belligerent sovereign is the judge of his own cause, and from such a judge we may hardly expect a measured and impartial judgment. Consequently, whether a war be truly just or unjust, once it is underway the armies on either side, following their respective princes, presumably fight in good faith, which means that they at least are convinced that their cause is just. "Assuming a demonstrable ignorance either of fact or of law," explains Victoria, "it may be that on the side where true justice is the war is just of itself, while on the other side the war is just in the sense of being excused from sin by reason of good faith, because invincible ignorance is a complete excuse."[19] In other words, impossible as it is in theory for the causes of both sides of a war to be just, in practice this is nearly always the case.[20] This fact, combined with Victoria's assertion that "in war everything is lawful which the defense of the common weal requires,"[21] to the "naked eye," as it were, most wars are just on both sides, at least once they are underway, and both armies may legitimately do what needs to be done to win. After all, though not to be found in either canon or civil law, everyone knows that the first law of war is to win, whatever it takes. We might well wonder whether

19. Victoria, *De Iure Belli*, 32.

20. This same point was later made more clearly by the eighteenth-century Swiss philosopher, diplomat, and legal scholar Emer de Vattel, when he wrote,

> War cannot be just on both sides. . . . It may however happen that both the contending parties are candid and sincere in their intentions; and, in a doubtful cause, it is still uncertain which side is in the right. Wherefore, since nations are equal and independent . . . and cannot claim a right of judgment over each other, it follows, that in every case susceptible of doubt, the arms of the two parties at war are to be accounted equally lawful, at least as to external effects, and until the decision of the cause. But neither does that circumstance deprive other nations of the liberty of forming their own judgment on the case, in order to determine how they are to act, and to assist that party who shall appear to have right on his side; nor does that effect of the independence of nations operate in exculpation of the author of an unjust war, who certainly incurs a high degree of guilt. But if he acts in consequence of invincible ignorance or error, the injustice of his arms is not imputable to him (*Law of Nations*, 39–40).

21. Victoria, *De Iure Belli*, 15.

Victoria would take serious issue with this claim, since with some doubts and reservations he accepts as legitimate in a just war such practices as the incidental slaughter of innocents, the summary execution of prisoners, the post-victory killing of guilty enemy combatants—especially non-Christians—and the enslavement of all enemy subjects, including women and children, guilty or not guilty, provided they be Saracens or other notorious pagans "of this type."[22]

After a thousand years, Christian just war theory—considering that the work of Franciscus de Victoria ranked as one of its high-water marks—was clearly a moral vessel with countless cracks in its hull. Surveying its history as we have, it is easy to forget and still easier to doubt that it served to limit the incidence and savagery of war, but admittedly we have no accurate means of imagining what even greater chaos might have occurred without it. That said, Erasmus was clearly convinced that the theory of just war, instead of thrusting a thumb in the dike, offered a thumbs up to war, and that the church had always had better things to do than to close its eyes and embrace it:

> Even if we allow that some wars are just, yet since we see that all mankind is plagued by this madness, it should be the role of wise priests to turn the minds of people and princes to other things. Nowadays we often see them as very firebrands of war. Bishops are not ashamed to frequent the camp; the cross is there, the body of Christ is there, the heavenly sacraments become mixed up in this worse than hellish business, and the symbols of perfect charity are brought into these bloody conflicts. Still more absurd, Christ is present in both camps, as if fighting against himself. It is not enough for war to be permitted between Christians; it must also be accorded the supreme honor.[23]

The last towering figure whose work we will consider here turned, or more properly scripted, a new page in the history of just war theory and international law. Hugo Grotius, a Dutch Protestant, a jurist by profession, brought to his work a vast learning of philosophy and the classics, together with a genuine horror at the violence of his times. "Throughout the Christian world," wrote Grotius, "I observed a lack of restraint in relation to war, such as even barbarous races should be ashamed of; I observed that men rush to arms for slight causes, or no causes at all."[24] So, the latest

22. Ibid., 32.
23. Erasmus, *Collected Works*, 27:108.
24. Grotius, *De Iure Belli*, vol. 3. Prolegomena to the First Edition, 28.

in a long line of those who would argue restraint in war, Grotius penned a massive three-volume treatise titled *De Iure Belli ac Pacis* (*The Rights of War and Peace*) that provided both a magisterial, systematic summation of the just war tradition to date and would become what many scholars came to acknowledge as the cornerstone of modern international law. Although Grotius, like his predecessors, was a committed Christian and drew freely from biblical, classical, and scholastic literature, unlike his predecessors his aim was to write a text that "would have a degree of validity even if we should concede that which cannot be conceded without the utmost wickedness—that there is no God or that the affairs of men are of no concern to him."[25]

In arguing for a valid law of nations, binding on all princes and polities, Grotius confronted a relatively new threat to the rule of morality and law posed by those who, like Machiavelli, denied the existence of any natural law or universal legal order. It was their contention that utility is the mother of justice and that nothing is unjust that is necessary or expedient. Grotius, like it or not, found himself required to give up considerable ground to those "realists" inasmuch as they read their times, as well as the future, with undeniable, if regrettable, accuracy. To try to hold them to a far higher standard than they would ever accept was pointless preaching to a choir that was no longer there. Instead, in the words of political scientist Steven Forde, Grotius

> attempted to define a theoretical position between an idealism he thought counterproductive and an amoral realism he found unacceptable. Grotius constructed a system in which the moral authority of natural law was combined with the flexibility of human law. This required him to develop a special understanding of the nature and relation of these two types of law. In giving the law of nations, as a product of human will, the authority to suspend provisions of natural law, he provided for a code of international conduct that could permit injustice where necessary, without abandoning moral ideals altogether.[26]

One of Grotius' core concessions was that natural law was obviously alterable, precisely because in the march of human civilization it had in fact been altered in fundamental ways and continued to evolve and mutate in response to human imagination and will. Natural law properly belonged to a primitive and pre-civil human condition that man had long since left

25. Ibid., 11.
26. Forde, "Hugo Grotius," 639.

behind in favor of civil law and the law of nations, which though rooted in natural law are morally compromised and permissive compared to the law that was first etched into our nature. Yielding to expedience, necessity, and human imperfection, civil or positive law is accustomed to granting certain exemptions from the prescriptions of natural law to allow such "unnatural" institutions as private property, slavery, and war. Human conventional law, then, taking form and operating by human compact, no longer represented for Grotius the simple implementation of natural law, as Aquinas and Suarez had understood it to be.

We need to be clear here, however, that when civil or international law amends natural law and grants permission for its violation, it does not make right what was wrong or make just what was unjust. It grants immunity not innocence, allowing an individual or a state to act wrongly or unjustly with impunity. But there are limits, as Grotius sees it, to the immunity from natural law that any human law can rightly offer. Human law, he asserts, cannot command what natural law prohibits, nor can it prohibit what natural law commands,[27] which at the same time means that it may permit whatever natural law forbids and decline to enforce whatever natural law enjoins.

What did all this mean, we rightly ask, for Grotius' views on war? In the first place it meant that he rejected pacifism out of hand as unrealistic and irrelevant. This despite the fact that he detested war and saw that no good could ever come from it. "War has no place," he wrote, "among the useful arts. Nay, rather, it is so horrible that only the utmost necessity, or true charity, can render it honourable."[28] What Grotius sought, however, were practical, effective moral and legal restraints on war and its horror, and he didn't see how these could ever come from the preaching of pacifism. In the judgment of Grotius, as summed up by Forde, the proponents of Christian nonviolence

> actually undermine the prospects for restraint by going too far in the opposite direction. Their extremism only discredits reasonable moral argument and robs morality of what effect it might have on practice. . . . Excessive idealism only marginalizes itself; a more responsible approach must begin by making peace with certain uncomfortable realities.[29]

27. See Grotius, *De Iure Belli*, II.2.5.
28. Ibid., II.10.9, 3.
29. Forde, "Hugo Grotius," 639.

Unfortunately, by Grotius' admission, the middle ground that he staked out between nonviolence and war without rules led to his making peace with a range of criminal behavior, on the grounds that the world was not yet ready for a higher standard. Better a base and broken standard than none at all, and from that beginning one can at least hope for and work towards a more just law of nations that will progressively minimize the savagery and suffering of war.

Grotius understood war in judicial terms. "It is evident," he explained, "that the sources from which wars arise are as numerous as those from which lawsuits spring; for where judicial settlement fails, war begins."[30] War represents, then, the resort to force when judicial means fail to resolve competing charges or claims. As in a judicial hearing or court case, each of the adversarial parties are to be granted their day in court, or in this case, their day on the field of battle. Grotius argued that according to the law of nations in any "public war," a war between sovereign states, it is permissible (setting aside whether it is just) for the armies of both sides to do lethal harm to each other, as well as to the legal subjects of both warring states, including infants and women, captives, those wishing to surrender, and those surrendering unconditionally. Regarding what level or kind of lethal harm may be done, he states that "in war things which are necessary to attain the end in view are permissible."[31] Amidst these and innumerable other rules of war discussed in *De Iure Belli ac Pacis,* one fact is lost on no one, least of all Grotius. Legal war is not and will likely never be just war. Grotius leaves his readers with no doubt that he was personally troubled and saddened by the low standard of conduct that legal war condones. In fact, he reminds them that there is a higher law that they could choose to follow, and he exhorts them to do so in these words:

> Many things are said to be "lawful," or "permissible" for the reason that they are done with impunity, in part also because coactive tribunals lend to them their authority; things which, nevertheless, either deviate from the rule of right (whether this has its basis in law strictly so called, or in the admonitions of other virtues), or at any rate may be omitted on higher grounds and with greater praise among good men.[32]

30. Grotius, *De Iure Belli,* II.1.2, 1.

31. Ibid., 3.1.2, 1.

32. Ibid., 3.23.1, 1

By the time Georg Friedrich von Martens published his *Precis du Droit des Gens de l'Europe* in 1789, nearly a century and a half after the death of Grotius in 1645, European common law had wholly eclipsed the last remnants of the just war tradition. Von Martens gave it no more than a brief mention and only so as to dismiss it. "In retrospect," wrote von Martens, "it appears that the traditional doctrine of just war is essentially religious; where its religious spirit evaporates, only a shallow and stale residue remains."[33] Commenting on von Martens' assessment of the just war tradition, Professor Arthur Nussbaum of Berlin University and the Academie de Droit International at the Hague writes,

> He [von Martens] points out that war, if not "manifestly unjust," is actually being considered by both parties as lawful in respect to the treatment of the enemy and the validity of conventions and treaties. This statement, reminiscent of Grotian tenets, has thenceforth never been questioned, except that the qualification regarding "manifest unjustness" has been abandoned. This evolution amounts to a universal recognition of the legal irrelevance of the just-war conception, especially if one adds the well-settled elimination of the latter from the law of neutrality.[34]

The essentially religious and ethical character of the just war tradition is also asserted by Josef Kunz, who reminds us of the obvious fact that "it is of Catholic origin, anchored in natural law, a theological, not a legal concept."[35] He goes on to make the more poignant case that "this doctrine in its purity, even if it might have been or were a norm of positive international law, would be practically valueless because of the grave objections against its workability. This very circumstance forced later writers to develop the doctrine in such a way as to deform it."[36] Indeed, we have traced its progressive deformation to the point that it provided no practical means for distinguishing just from unjust war and granted so many decisive immunities and permissions that it condoned what we today would without hesitation label as war crimes. Frederick Russell, in an effort to sum up and assess the legacy of the just war tradition, has this to say:

> For the past 3000 years, just war theories have had the dual purpose of restraining and justifying violence, essentially a

33. Martens, *Précis du Droit*, 478.
34. Nussbaum, "Just War," 42.
35. Kunz, "Bellum Justum," 530.
36. Ibid., 531.

self-contradictory exercise. Either the just war was a moral and religious doctrine, in which it was deprived of coercive but not normative force, or it was a legal concept that served as a cloak for statism. It remains an open question whether just war theories have limited more wars than they have encouraged.[37]

Remarkably and with presumably good intentions, centuries after its obituary had been filed, there was a concerted effort to resuscitate just war theory following World War I, and the result is that it has haunted political and moral discourse and debate for the past century. During that time, the concept of just war has been invoked to drape with legitimacy every major war that the United States has waged and is waging since that time, despite the fact that none of these conflicts would have met the criteria for just war before those criteria became so opportunistically diluted and distorted that they could be used to stamp as legitimate whatever acts a warring nation deems necessary to prevail, such as the firebombing of civilian populations in Europe and Southeast Asia, the dropping of the first nuclear weapons in Japan, the "shock and awe" devastation of Baghdad, and the unleashing of a growing squadron of predator drones for purposes of assassination and terror in countries with whom we are not formally at war. If just war doctrine ever served to limit more chaos and suffering than it licensed, which is ever so questionable, it has long since abandoned that function. If there is a better way to leash the dogs of war, the time has surely come to find it.

37. Russell, *Just War*, 308.

8

Conclusion

Beyond Just War

J UST WAR THEORY IS a dead letter. This is the argument advanced, if not
proven, in the preceding chapters. It was never more than a theory,
and at its worst it was a lie, a deadly lie. It promised at least the possibility
of war without sin, war without criminality, war without guilt or shame,
war in which men would risk their lives but not their souls. At its headi-
est, it promised war in which men would win eternal life, and now, in the
fullness of wartime, these same promises have been extended to women.
Whether or not these promises were first or ever made in good faith is
something we can never know, and it doesn't matter. What we can know is
that they have not been kept. We know this from experience, the experience of war, the killing lab in which the theory of just war has been tested
for sixteen centuries. It is time to declare its death and to write an autopsy.

Some moments, in retrospect, decide everything. When the two most
towering minds and influential thinkers in the history of Western Christianity came to the conclusion that not all killing was murder and that not
all wars were evil, they sealed away in silence one of the most profound
and potentially transformative bits of "good news" at the core of that very
faith to which they had confessedly dedicated their lives—that love is more
powerful than hate and that it is better to die than to kill. They and those
who followed them came to see the pacifism of the early church as mere
"passivism," as doing nothing, as unrealistic, naive, and irresponsible. In

arming Christians for righteous battle, they disarmed the radical challenge and alternative to war embodied in the early Christian community, whose own "heroes" gave their lives as willingly as any warriors, while refusing to take the lives of others.

Despite the official ecclesiastical adoption of just war, however, the Christian community has never spoken with one voice regarding war. There have always been those often lone and marginalized doubters and resisters who have questioned and decried the church's long affair with the god of war. In our own day, one of those voices of dissent is Daniel Berrigan, a Jesuit priest who has relentlessly confronted his country and his church with their complicity in the lethal illusion of just war. As he sees it,

> It came to something like this. . . . One could undergo, as [others] had undergone, and their parents before them, the entire Christian induction, the seasonal rhythms of Christian worship, could receive the Christian sacraments; could be exposed year after year to elite Christian education. And still one would go off to war, in apparent good conscience.
>
> In the course of the war, any war, vast numbers of the enemy, whether combatants or bystanders or the ill or aged or newly born, would be disposed of by slaughterhouse technique. There would occur also vast numbers of casualties on one's own side.
>
> And all this would be wrought and undergone in truly awesome good faith; a faith shored up and accompanied by the church's blessing.
>
> Further; this increasingly lax conscience with regard to mass murder—this could be expanded until it encompassed all the living. There would be no limits established, no end in sight. The nature of state violence was illimitable; persuasive reasons would be adduced for ending the human venture.
>
> Nor would any limit be set by the church.[1]

And yet "just war" was from the beginning supposed to mean "limited war." This was the explicit intent of its founding fathers and erstwhile advocates. But intentions, as we have seen, are for God's eyes only. Everyone else is left to stare at and live with the consequences. And in this case the consequences have overstepped every limit imaginable, save human extinction, which we have risked and to which we have come perilously close.

Christian theologians and canon lawyers, from Ambrose to Victoria, acknowledged that war, even just war, is fraught with matters of conscience,

1. Berrigan, *To Dwell in Peace*, 108.

claiming that the church, its clergy, and ultimately its pope are the proper and privileged adjudicators of such matters. Surely the history of "just" or "limited" war, however, has subverted that claim. The church's longstanding obsession with sexuality and complacency with war—still in evidence today—have all but disqualified the clergy and its hierarchy as the church's conscience in matters of making love and making war. Their canonical exclusion from the marriage bed and the battlefield has rendered most Catholic celibate clerics, past and present, personally inexperienced and professionally dubious as moral guides in those turbulent territories. Better to make a fresh start and to listen to those who know firsthand what they are talking about. When the reality in question is war, this means that we would do best to listen long and hard to combat veterans, as well as the correspondents who take notes at their side. In what follows now, we will make a start at doing just that.

"The idea that there are rules in warfare," wrote Sebastian Junger, after spending fifteen months embedded with a single platoon at a remote outpost in the Korangal Valley of Afghanistan, "and that combatants kill each other according to the basic concepts of fairness probably ended for good with the machine gun."[2] In fact, that particular idea must have ended much sooner, perhaps when mounted knights fell prey to the longbow or when the warriors of Asia first faced the Greek phalanx. Regardless, Junger's observation is that "soldiers gravitate toward whatever works best with the least risk," and

> At that point combat stops being a grand chess game between generals and becomes a no-holds-barred experiment in pure killing. As a result, much of modern military tactics is geared toward maneuvering the enemy into a position where they can essentially be massacred from safety. It sounds dishonorable only if you imagine that modern war is about honor; it's not. It's about winning, which means killing the enemy on the most unequal terms possible. Anything less simply results in the loss of more of your own men.[3]

In other words, combat is about killing without dying, however that can best be accomplished, whether with an ambush, an artillery barrage, a high-altitude bombing mission, or a predator drone. If this was ever not the case, that memory is all but lost and has no influence on policy or practice today. On paper, just war was to be all about proportionality and fair play.

2. Junger, *War*, 140.
3. Ibid.

What made it irrelevant was that it just didn't describe war. War has its own rules, and they don't include fair play, moral limits, or an agreement that right trumps might. War, as Bertrand Russell is said to have once memorably stated, never decides who's right, just who's left. It is, as Vietnam veteran William Mahedy put it, "a moral sewer"[4] that can't be cleaned up and whose waters never were and never will be morally potable.

Perhaps the most impressive and touted secular heir to the just war tradition's dream of limited warfare is the Geneva Conventions, as Gary D. Solis, retired Professor of Law at the U.S. Military Academy, argues:

> The 1949 Geneva Conventions are the cornerstone of the law of war. They are the most adhered-to treaties in history. Every nation in the world has ratified them. . . . The 1949 Conventions have stood the test of more than 60 years of armed conflicts, revolutions, civil wars, rebellions, and insurgencies. Yes, there are some odd provisions contained in the 429 Articles of the four 1949 Conventions. The Conventions nevertheless remain the most significant brake on the horrors of warfare, and the most significant protector of victims of war that a compassionate world can devise.[5]

Even a quick backward glance, however, over the past six decades since the signing of the Conventions, raises obvious and troubling questions: What might it mean to say that "these are the most adhered-to treaties in history"? Does "adhered-to" mean anything more than merely "adopted" or "ratified"? To sign onto the Conventions is a far cry from observing them. In which of the more than eighty major armed conflicts waged since 1949 by treaty signatories were the Geneva Conventions not flagrantly violated? The French-Algerian War? Vietnam? The Soviet invasion of Afghanistan? The Iraq-Iran War? The civil wars in Sudan and Rwanda? The Arab-Israeli Wars? Kosovo? Operation Iraqi Freedom? If the Conventions have indeed succeeded in "standing the test" of these years and their wars, what would all-out failure have looked like? In the face of the many tens of millions slaughtered in these conflicts—the vast majority of them noncombatants—how can anyone take heart or find hope in the knowledge that the Conventions "remain the most significant brake on the horrors of warfare, and the most significant protector of victims of war that a compassionate world can devise"?

The Geneva Conventions, as we know, have not been alone in their concern for the humane treatment of war prisoners and for the protection

4. Mahedy, *Out of the Night*, 101.

5. *Geneva Conventions* 1–2.

of noncombatants. A range of other authorities and institutions are determined to police or limit war, such as the United Nations and the International Criminal Court, and these often focus on the prevention and punishment of war crimes and crimes against humanity. For all its good intent and occasional achievement, what this focus misses, however, is the essential and thus inescapable criminality and atrocity of all war. Lawyers, like the theologians that preceded them, are often too quick to believe that the distinctions and rules they inscribe in their documents will have any ordering or taming effect on the chaos of war. What must be said again and again until it sinks in is that war has its own rules, and they have little or nothing to do with serving justice or preserving humanity.

Casting our eyes and our questions closer to home, we may well ask how well the United States has "stood the test" of putting the brake on the horrors of warfare and protecting innocent civilians. Robert McNamara—an Army Air Forces officer in our "best" war and Secretary of Defense during arguably our "worst" war—had ample cause and opportunity for reflecting on the rules of war. When asked about the firebombing of Tokyo and other Japanese cities, including the incineration of one hundred thousand Japanese civilians in a single night, he admitted that "proportionality should be a guideline in war" and that

> Killing 50% to 90% of the people of 67 Japanese cities and then bombing them with two nuclear bombs is not proportional, in the minds of some people, to the objectives we were trying to achieve. . . .
>
> What one can criticize is that the human race prior to that time and today has not really grappled with what are, I'll call it, "the rules of war." Was there a rule then that said you shouldn't bomb, shouldn't kill, shouldn't burn to death 100,000 civilians in one night?[6]

The answer, of course, was that yes, there was a rule that you shouldn't slaughter civilians. And, apparently unbeknownst to McNamara, the human race had been grappling with the rules of war for millennia. But the truth was, and he knew it, the rules don't matter, not for winners. With remarkable candor McNamara related that Major General Curtis LeMay, who in the last year of the war directed all the strategic bombing missions against the Japanese home islands and under whom Lieutenant Colonel McNamara then served, confessed that, "If we'd lost the war, we'd all have

6. Morris, *Fog of War*, transcript.

been prosecuted as war criminals." In fact, LeMay had fully expected to be prosecuted as a war criminal after the war and McNamara agreed with his assessment:

> I think he's right. He, and I'd say I, were behaving as war criminals. LeMay recognized that what he was doing would be thought immoral if his side had lost. But what makes it immoral if you lose and not immoral if you win?[7]

The lesson that McNamara says he learned from his war experience is that "in order to do good, you may have to engage in evil . . . But how much evil," he asks, "must we do in order to do good?" Judging from his service in World War II and later his presiding over the Vietnam War, we might find that evil to be incalculable.

In U.S. military policy limited warfare has come to mean at least two things: limited in duration and limited in U.S. and allied casualties. The other side of this coin is unlimited force. Joint Vision 2010, described by General John M. Shalikashvili, then Chairman of the Joint Chiefs of Staff, as "an operationally based template for the evolution of the Armed Forces for a challenging and uncertain future,"[8] calls for "full spectrum dominance"[9] and on every level of combat "an order of magnitude improvement in lethality."[10] In a world where the United States sees "American global hegemony" as "the West's last hope for survival,"[11] "there is still no substitute for victory."[12] All future wars must be "short and decisive—with success measured entirely in the destruction of enemy forces."[13] Regrettably, the destruction of enemy forces will all but inevitably entail a far greater destruction of civilian infrastructure and population, but if McNamara is right, so long as we are victorious we will never be seen, much less prosecuted, as criminals.

Today, the operative rules of war for our boots-on-the-ground troops in Iraq and Afghanistan are called the ROE, the Rules of Engagement, dictating when and how much force is authorized and appropriate in any given

7. Ibid.
8. Shalikashvili, *Joint Vision 2010*, front matter.
9. Ibid., 2.
10. Ibid., 13.
11. Linn, "U.S. Armed Forces' View," 37.
12. Nagl, "Let's Win," 26.
13. Ibid., 38.

situation. In today's war zones, the ROE are the only limits in place. But how well do they work? After three deployments in Iraq between 2003 and 2006, Marine Sergeant Jason Wayne Lemieux offers this assessment:

> In general, the Rules of Engagement changed frequently and were contradictory. When they were restrictive, they were loosely enforced. Shootings of civilians that were known were not reported because marines did not want to send their brothers-in-arms to prison when all they were trying to do was protect themselves in a situation they'd been forced into. With no way to identify their attackers, and no clear mission worth dying for, marines viewed the Rules of Engagement as either a joke or a technicality to be worked around so that they could bring each other home alive. Not only are the misuses of the Rules of Engagement in Iraq indicative of supreme strategic incompetence, they are also a moral disgrace. The people who set them should be ashamed of themselves.[14]

Marine Corporal Jason Washburn, also with three Iraq deployments behind him, recalls how in his experience the ROE governing the identification of combatants and the recognition of threat were regularly bent and broken so as to bestow virtual impunity on him and his fellow Marines:

> Something else we were encouraged to do, almost with a wink and nudge, was to carry drop weapons, or by my third tour, drop shovels. We would carry these weapons or shovels with us because if we accidentally shot a civilian, we could just toss the weapon on the body, and make them look like an insurgent. By my third tour, we were told that if they carried a shovel or a heavy bag, or if they were seen digging anywhere, especially near roads, that we could shoot them. So we carried these tools and weapons in our vehicles in case we accidentally shot an innocent civilian. We could just toss it on there and be like, "Well, he was digging. I was within the Rules of Engagement." This was commonly encouraged, but only behind closed doors. There obviously wasn't a public announcement, but it was pretty common.[15]

Lastly, to highlight further the extent to which our troops in Iraq were made or at least left to operate without any operative moral compass, there is this report from Army Specialist Hart Viges, who served in Iraq in 2003–4:

14. Glantz, *Winter Soldier*, 19.
15. Ibid., 22.

> And the radio—a good thing never came over the radio. One time they said to fire on all taxi cabs because the enemy was using them for transportation. In Iraq, any car can be a taxi cab; you just paint it white and orange. One of the snipers replied back, "Excuse me? Did I hear that right? Fire on all taxi cabs?" The lieutenant colonel responded, "You heard me, trooper, fire on all taxi cabs." After that, the town lit up, with all the units firing on cars. This was my first experience with war, and that kind of set the tone for the rest of the deployment.[16]

Ex-Marine Lieutenant Karl Marlantes poignantly relates how, when he raised his right hand in 1964, swore an oath to obey the Commander in Chief, and signed up with the Marine Corps, he in his own words "believed that a president of the United States would never give men an order that would cause any moral conflict."[17] His service in Vietnam, where he won the Navy Cross, two Navy Commendation Medals, two Purple Hearts, and ten Air Medals, was marked with distinction. It also, by his own account, left him haunted: "The Marine Corps taught me to kill but it didn't teach me how to deal with killing."[18] War is all about killing. "I think it's fair to say," writes ex-Marine Captain and Iraq veteran Tyler Boudreau,

> that the taking of human life is something we, as a species, are inherently reluctant to do. I've read that in books, but I've felt it in my gut too. But the soldier kills for a living—it is his reason for being. Killing is not a by-product or some shitty collateral duty like peeling potatoes or scrubbing the latrine. It is the institutional point. It's not a trade secret. It just is.
>
> And when a Marine shoots better than his peers, he's admired and he's handed medals and badges and promotions—all to encourage him to pull the trigger with another man in his sights and kill him. Like it or not, that's desensitization. But desensitization doesn't eliminate morality from the consciousness. It merely postpones cogitation. Sooner or later, when a man's had a chance to think things over, he will find himself standing in judgment before his own conscience.
>
> General Mattis, who'd been my Division Commander in Iraq, was once quoted: "It's fun to shoot some people . . . it's a hoot." The media went crazy. They splashed the quote all over the place. People were appalled. The papers described him as a monster.

16. Ibid., 55–56.
17. Marlantes, *What It Is Like*, 134.
18. Ibid., 3.

That was an odd reaction, I thought. Nobody in the Marine Corps was ruffled, not even the Commandant. And that's because in the Corps everyone gets it. Marines know that you say what you've got to say to make men kill, and to make yourself kill. Everybody does it from Private to General—all the time. Mattis' only mistake, I suppose, was sharing it with the public.[19]

Sooner or later there comes a time for, in Boudreau's words, "cogitation" and "standing in judgment before [one's] own conscience." Sometimes this painful interior rendezvous comes after years of denial and inner flight, but it can also break in today or tomorrow with unexpected suddenness and speed. Soldiers who one day have no questions or qualms about their duties, can the next day find themselves frozen stiff by a command or situation, once familiar but now quite foreign and paralyzing. Some call this the "crystallization of conscience."[20] Others call it a damned nuisance. Whatever we call it or however we understand it, such a moment of moral crisis is all too real. It demands a response and sends many soldiers looking for counsel. For many, the obvious or only place to find it is the chaplain. But appealing to military chaplains for moral guidance in war can be a disillusioning experience. It certainly was for Sergeant Ricky Clousing, an army interrogator in Iraq, who was shocked and confused to find his fellow soldiers pillaging Iraqi homes and hauling back the loot—televisions, cash, jewelry, and electronic equipment—to their barracks. Far worse still was when his staff sergeant posted two men at the door of an Iraqi home and raped a fourteen- or fifteen-year-old girl inside. Seeking out assistance from counselors and chaplains proved futile, as they "seemed more interested in stifling his misgivings than considering them."[21] So, as he put it, "I just kind of hit a brick wall and didn't know where to go":[22]

> I mean, I guess I was asking pretty big questions. But I was just wanting to find some answers. . . . I went and talked with the chaplains and told them about the spiritual basis for my conflict of conscience. They came back with all these cliché statements, and even Bible verses taken out of context, justifying war and saying God is favoring us, and that I should just trust in his plan. Just

---

19. Boudreau, *Packing Inferno*, 78, 81–82.

20. See the Truth Commission on Conscience in War at http://conscienceinwar.org.

21. Gutmann and Lutz, *Breaking Ranks*, 120.

22. Ibid.

> surfacey, watered-down statements that didn't answer anything that I was really feeling.
>
> I was reading the Bible and finding a lot of scriptures that were showing me a different side of Christianity, primarily about being peacemakers. The verses about love your neighbor as thyself, those who live by the sword die by the sword. I was going to Bible study for a while, but I stopped going because I didn't feel like I fit in, it wasn't comfortable. The chaplain was praying before missions that we would be God's hand of justice, and all the guys around me were bowing their heads and praying for this when forty minutes before they were watching porno on their computers and laughing about shooting animals.[23]

In December 1968, Karl Marlantes experienced a similar disillusionment on a mountaintop near the border of North and South Vietnam. He and his company of three Marine platoons had suffered soul-splitting casualties and were dead weary in spirit. "I was afraid I would die," remembers Marlantes:

> I held the lives of others in my hands. I had entered the temple of Mars, where not only were humans sacrificed, including me, but I was also the priest. This priest, however, had only been to a seminary called the Basic School where he had learned the ritual moves but none of the meaning.[24]

Then, two days before Christmas, when the fog lifted long enough to allow a single supply helicopter to reach them, it came complete with a real priest aboard, the battalion chaplain. Marlantes remembers him and that moment well:

> He had brought with him several bottles of Southern Comfort and some new dirty jokes. I accepted the Southern Comfort, thanked him, laughed at the jokes, and had a drink with him. Merry Christmas.
>
> Inside I was seething. I thought I'd gone a little nuts. How could I be angry with a guy who had just put his life at risk to cheer me up? And didn't the Southern Comfort feel good on that rain-raked mountaintop? Years later I understood. I was engaged in killing and maybe being killed. I felt responsible for the lives and deaths of my companions. I was struggling with a situation approaching the sacred in its terror and contact with the infinite,

23. Ibid., 121.
24. Marlantes, *What It Is Like*, 5.

and he was trying to numb me to it. I needed help with the existential terror of my own death and responsibility for the death of others, enemies and friends, not Southern Comfort. I needed a spiritual guide.[25]

To be sure, not all military chaplains are cheerleaders and some are able to offer a good deal more wisdom than can be found in a bottle of bourbon. But from all I have read and heard from veterans of recent wars, they are not the rule. The late Reverend William Mahedy, a chaplain in Vietnam and then, for the rest of his remarkable life, a VA and Vet Center counselor, was one of the exceptions. Even so, he accepted responsibility, along with his fellow chaplains, for what he saw as their failure in Vietnam. More specifically, their failure "to discern the moral and religious meaning of what was taking place. The men, both as soldiers during their combat and as veterans, after the war, have been looking for moral guidance and spiritual direction, but they have received neither."[26]

In part, Mahedy blames the training he and other chaplains received both as seminarians and later during their basic officer course and in various chaplain seminars, all of which he describes as a "virtual orgy" of group dynamics and sensitivity sessions, all about caring and affirming, while meanwhile evading real moral and religious issues. "I believe the essential failure of the chaplaincy in Vietnam," explains Mahedy,

> was its inability to name the reality for what it was. We should first have called it sin, admitted we were in a morally ambiguous and religiously tenuous situation, and then gone on to deal with the harsh reality of the soldier's life. . . . In theological terms, war is sin. This has nothing to do with whether a particular war is justified or whether isolated incidents in a soldier's war were right or wrong. The point is that war as a human enterprise is a matter of sin. It is a form of hatred for one's fellow human beings. It produces alienation from others and nihilism, and it ultimately represents a turning away from God.[27]

Ironically, a military chaplain is often in no good position to do anything but evade the real moral and religious issues of war. True enough, he is "a man of the cloth," but the cloth in this case is a military uniform. On the left collar of his battle fatigues is a cross or other religious insignia, but

25. Ibid., 7.
26. Mahedy, *Out of the Night*, 133.
27. Ibid., 135, 115.

across from it on his right shoulder is an insignia indicating his military rank. As Mahedy explains, "He is, like the soldiers themselves and their military commanders, an integral part of the 'green machine,' the army":

> He is seen as inseparable from the basic function of the green machine, which is killing. In our previous wars, no one questioned the relationship between the religious and military roles of chaplains. The reason, of course, is that in previous wars there was little doubt in anyone's mind that the fight was a noble sacrifice of almost religious dimensions. *Pro Deo et Patria* (For God and Country), the motto of the Army Chaplain Corps, was accepted as entirely appropriate because there was no perceived disjunction between the intention of God and the American cause.[28]

Although the harmonious marriage of God and country fell on rocky times during the sixties and seventies, the union survived and in the eyes of most Americans, God and country are once again a happy couple. The ever-growing influence, even predominance, of Christian evangelicals in the military hierarchy, including the Chaplain Corps, particularly in the army and the air force, all but assures the theological and political future and vitality of our national civic religion, with its core belief in predestined American exceptionalism. To put it mildly, writes Mahedy,

> The notion of war as sin simply doesn't play in Peoria—or anywhere else in the United States—because a fondness for war is an essential component of the macho American god. We define deity as that supreme being who achieves his ends by force. In our cultural definition of God, his divine purposes and our national goals are coextensive. The nation is the agent by which God works his will in the world. The means by which these purposes are realized is force. Given these assumptions, it is extraordinarily difficult to conduct a public discussion of war as sin. Yet the awareness of evil—in religious terms a consciousness of sin—is the underlying motif of the Vietnam War stories.[29]

And, we might add, of the war stories coming out of Iraq and Afghanistan.

The American myth—that we are a nation under God, stamped with his seal of approval, gifted with a unique destiny, and carrying a lifetime guarantee on our wars, that they will be just and successful—is alive and well, at least in the public sphere. No one running for office, mounting a

28. Ibid., 132.
29. Ibid., 155.

pulpit, or wearing a uniform can challenge it without paying a high price for his or her blasphemy. The sacred mask of American mythology, however, can't help but slip in war, and reveal to those close at hand the true face behind it. A nation at war is never a nation under God. When this truth sinks in, combat soldiers and vets often enter what Mahedy has called "a bleak and painful dark night of the spirit," and it is the responsibility of the church to go there with them:

> Greater exposure to the spiritual sufferings of the vets should bring about within the Church a recognition that the dark night of the soul is an authentic Christian mystical experience. The American Church has evaded the dark night through near-total immersion in a culture that seeks personal and national well-being at the expense of every other value.[30]

Listening to our vets may well prove to be a conversion experience for the American church, no less momentous than the conversion of Augustine, the father of the just war tradition. His story is well known, how he heard the voice of a boy in a nearby garden singing *tolle et lege*, "take and read," and so he did—closing his eyes, opening his Bible, and pointing to a passage to which he opened his soul as if it had come directly from the mouth of God. Today, there are other young "boys" (and women) asking the church to *sedere et audire*, to sit and listen to them, their stories, their confusion, guilt, and shame. Their voices too might come from God, who is known to speak in unexpected and unwelcome ways.

It is today's combat veterans who are bringing the greatest clarity to the moral cost of any war. They know as well as anyone else and better than most that we live in a violent world and that neither we nor those who threaten us are likely to lay down arms anytime soon, making war as a last resort necessary in the extreme. That said, they are far less likely than most of us to concede that a war of necessity is by definition a just war. In fact, many of them have begun to ask themselves and their country whether there is any such thing as a just war. After all, it is our veterans who have lived and endured the inescapable contradiction between the touted necessity of violence and its inherent immorality. The nation that sent them to war sees them as heroes, deserving our lasting gratitude and esteem; but all too often they return from war unable to accept that gratitude and respect, finding themselves inwardly darkened and eaten away with guilt and shame. This reality is something we all need to understand,

30. Ibid., 189.

and this understanding will never come unless we listen to our veterans and learn from them, rather than from our political representatives and leaders, about the "rules of war"—referred to as the "rules of the road" by our president in his Nobel Peace Prize acceptance speech—and whether they matter for much in the end.

Here we find ourselves again where our discussion of moral injury began, with combat veterans who have followed all the rules and find themselves lost. Some speak of having lost their humanity, while others express the fear that they have lost their souls. Like Septimus Warren Smith, the shadowed and shattered veteran of the Great War in Virginia Woolf's *Mrs. Dalloway*, they say, at least to themselves, "I have committed a crime."[31] And many like Septimus, unable to live with their pain, take their own lives. It may be that they are unable to convince themselves any longer that killing in war is any different from other kinds of killing. War "alters the dimensions of morality within a man's consciousness," explains Tyler Boudreau,

> and what is clearly wrong on the home front becomes natural on the battlefield. Killing, for instance, is a sin, unless you're in war, unless your life is threatened. Shooting an unarmed man is generally considered wrong, even in war, unless you think he's maneuvering against you. Then it's okay. Firing on the wounded or surrendered is not allowed, unless you believe they're faking. Then, by all means, fire away. So there are exceptions to the rules. That's what you pick up in the combat zone, the exceptions. The lines of morality shift and fade away, and so the soldier often doesn't even realize it's happening.[32]

Boudreau goes on to explain how warriors learn to handle this shifting moral terrain:

> Soldiers desensitize themselves in war, all in their own ways, but they all do it because they know that they must in order to survive, to push through the killing and to accomplish the mission, whatever the mission may be. They push the humanity out of the enemy and out of themselves and soon become mere bodies of instinct and survival. What is often discovered only later, sometimes too late, is that one's humanity can be quite difficult to recover once it's been evicted.[33]

---

31. Woolf, *Mrs. Dalloway*, 66.
32. Boudreau, *Packing Inferno*, 165.
33. Ibid., 83.

"Truth likes to hide,"[34] wrote the Greek philosopher Heraclitus, and no truth likes to do so quite as much as the truth of war. But the truth will and does come out. That "war is hell" is a truism. The full truth, though, is that war is hell not because it is a place of physical torment but because it is a place of distilled evil. Albert Camus, no theologian, reached the same conclusion after World War II. He saw the justification of murder as our most profound and consequential failing. He disallowed any distinction between killing and murder and argued that killing, even in self-defense, is never innocent, never without violation.[35] "It should break your heart to kill,"[36] writes veteran and poet Brian Turner. And it does. Taking a life breaks the heart and darkens the soul. Virtually every ancient and traditional society from India to Greece to Native America, however warlike, knew this. Our veterans know this. It is time for us as a nation to acknowledge it and to learn the rules of another road, the road to healing, and sooner rather than later the road to peace.

Commanders-in-chief of nations routinely and rightly acknowledge the grave responsibility and burden of sending others into harm's way, but never have I heard mention of the full extent of that potential harm. Life, limbs, and wits—physical and psychological well-being—are all openly at risk; but soul injury and death never come to mind or speech, except afterwards, and then mostly in closed circles. One notable exception was when former Senator Bob Kerrey, a Navy Seal in Vietnam, confessed that "I thought dying for your country was the worst thing that could happen to you, and I don't think it is. I think killing for your country can be a lot worse. Because that's the memory that haunts."[37] It is imperative for us to ponder these words, to listen to our veterans, to stop using the convenient rhetoric of just wars, and to heal the wounded and the haunted.

To set aside the rhetoric of just wars is, of course, itself no more than an exercise in honesty. It is simply to tell the truth about war, starting with our wars. But telling the truth is better than lying, and that is a step forward, a first step beyond war. We are a fearful nation in a fearful world. We fear others and they fear us even more. We even fear ourselves. Until we can confront our fear rather than succumb to it, we will never be able even to conceive of a world without war, much less embrace it. And the first fear

34. *phusis kruptesthai philei.* Heraclitus, fragment 123.
35. This is the central argument of *The Rebel.*
36. Turner, *Here, Bullet,* 56.
37. Quoted in MacNair, *Perpetration-Induced Traumatic Stress,* 167.

we must overcome on this road is the fear of the "other," each other. "The years we have gone through," wrote Camus after World War II, "have killed something in us. And that something is simply the old confidence man had in himself, which led him to believe that he could always elicit human reactions from another man if he spoke to him in the language of a common humanity."[38] Camus, who lost his father in the Battle of the Somme and was himself a core member of the French Resistance, struggled with fear and hatred, violence and nonviolence, throughout his life, and at one point after the liberation of Paris advocated the execution of France's most notorious collaborators. But in the end he convinced himself, and tried his best to convince others, that murder—never just or legitimate—is "a desperate exception or it is nothing."[39] He saw war too as a desperate exception, not the rule, not the natural condition of humankind, as so many would claim. "People like me," he explained,

> want not a world in which murder no longer exists (we are not so crazy as that!) but rather one in which murder is not legitimate. Here indeed we are Utopian—and contradictory. For we do live, it is true, in a world where murder is legitimate, and we ought to change it if we do not like it. . . . All I ask is that, in the midst of a murderous world, we agree to reflect on murder and to make a choice.[40]

The choice Camus had in mind was hope—hope in the fundamental decency and good will of humankind, hope in our essential solidarity, hope in what he saw as the human consortium of the damned, mortals doomed to die but not doomed to die at one another's hands. His voice will likely sound quite childish and hollow, of course, to ears long since bent and persuaded by more "realistic" words like these, from none other than Freud:

> Men are not gentle creatures who want to be loved, and who at the most can defend themselves if they are attacked; they are, on the contrary, creatures among whose instinctual endowments is to be reckoned a powerful share of aggressiveness. As a result, their neighbor is for them not only a potential helper or sexual object, but also someone who tempts them to satisfy their aggressiveness on him, to exploit his capacity for work without compensation, to use him sexually without his consent, to seize his possessions, to

38. Camus, *Neither Victims nor Executioners*, 1.
39. Camus, *Rebel*, 282.
40. Camus, *Neither Victims nor Executioners*, 4, 18.

humiliate him, to cause him pain, to torture and to kill him. *Homo homini lupus.* [Man is a wolf to man.] Who, in the face of all his experience of life and of history, will have the courage to dispute this assertion?[41]

In truth, what Freud describes here is not "reality" but a choice. And so with Augustine's "original sin" and Hobbes' "war of all against all" and all of the countless bleak diagnoses of our perverse and violent nature we know so well. Plato, I believe, was nearer the reality of our condition when he suggested that human beings span a vast moral universe of possibilities stretching from the heights to the depths, from the angelic to the demonic:

> Now man we call a gentle [*hemeron*] creature, but in truth, though he is wont to prove more god-like and gentle [*teiotaton hemerota-ton*] than any if he have but the right native endowments and the right schooling; let him be trained insufficiently or amiss, and he will show himself more savage [*agriotaton*] than anything on the face of the earth.[42]

Freud was right that it will take courage, in the face of our experience of life and history, to rear and educate our children to see their fellow citizens and human beings, not as predators or prey, but as they would themselves in a mirror, with hope and good will. As it is, our general education or "training" is ingenuous and unfair, in every sense of that word. In the United States, 99 percent of our population can at least pretend to be tame and gentle because they have outsourced their wilder, more fearful and violent impulses to the 1 percent of the population (the military and the police) who keep them safe by wielding whatever force is required to accomplish that. Whenever crime or war breaks out, or simply when night falls, the 99 percent take to their houses and lock the doors. Lethal force is only three numbers away, at their fingertips. True enough, as a last resort, nearly half of the 99 percent, hedging their bets, have armed themselves, and keep their own vigil. They know how to fire their weapons but few will ever take a human life with them. They, like the rest of us, leave that to our police and, most especially, to our armed services. But, if we are honest with ourselves, as Marine veteran Karl Marlantes reminds us, we already know that "killing people with Marines is ethically no different from killing

41. Freud, *Civilization and Its Discontents*, 58.
42. Plato, *Laws* 766a.

people with hatchets. Only the distance from the spurting blood differs."[43] Our "armed services" are, as their title suggests, our servants, our agents, our arms. We employ, commission, commend, and reward them for what they do on our behalf. They do for us what we want done but don't have the training or the inclination to do for ourselves. They have been "basically trained" to suspect, to hate, and to kill on impulse. And then they "graduate" to actual combat where they complete their education:

> Basic training is oriented toward eliminating the enemy's humanity.[44]

> There's always a lot of talk about developing hatred when it comes to war. You've got to hate them before you can kill them . . . that sort of thing.[45]

> Professional officers consider part of the psychological training of their troops to be training in hatred, and this becomes more systematized and subtler as the war goes on.[46]

There are many things desperately wrong with the fact that actually less than 1 percent of the population of the United States bear the full burden of learning to hate and kill their fellow human beings and not infrequently of actually doing so, while wagering not only their lives but also their souls in the bargain. First, it is unfair. Second, it removes the rest of us, the 99 percent, from the reality of war and allows us to imagine that we have not, at one remove, also grown accustomed to suspicion and hatred and learned to nod our approval at the deaths of other human beings, well over 90 percent of them civilians like ourselves, who do not and never would threaten us. When we care less about the deaths of others' children than we do about our own, as we read in the Hindu epic the *Mahabharata*, war is near. In that case, we live out our days on the brink. Third, our remove from war permits our leaders, while we sleep, to wage war with greater and greater ferocity and abandon, so that when we awake we find ourselves in a war without end and without limits.

This is where we find ourselves, in an age of endless war waged by our proxies, who in some cases are also our brothers and sisters, sons and daughters, fathers and mothers, and they are coming home to us shredded,

43. Marlantes, *What It Is Like*, 227.

44. Ibid., 232.

45. Boudreau, *Packing Inferno*, 75.

46. Gray, *Warriors*, 161.

when they come home at all. Yes, it will require rare courage for us, individually and as a nation, to choose a different path. In the end, I would suggest, that path must lead beyond war. For now, however, it is difficult for us even to imagine a world without war; and, supposing we could, how would we convince others to live in our imagined world? The answer can only be "one step at a time." With this in mind, I will conclude here by hazarding a few brief, concrete, and surely controversial suggestions as food for thought.

In the first place I would suggest that we call an end to our nation's four-decades-long experiment with an all-volunteer army. Granted, the Pentagon and defense establishment see this experiment as a smashing success and warn that we could never have fought our recent wars—nor can we fight our future wars—without an all-volunteer professional force. But this is precisely the point. These wars have been ill-conceived and have undermined the moral and economic integrity of our country; and the future wars we might imagine are still more frightening.

It is instructive and intriguing that a brilliant military historian, Theodore Fehrenbach, writing a half-century ago, well before the creation of our all-volunteer army, read our military future with remarkable prescience, predicting the creation of such a force and suggesting what it would mean for future warfare. "However repugnant the idea is to liberal societies," wrote Fehrenbach,

> the man who will willingly defend the free world in the fringe areas is not the responsible citizen-soldier. The man who will go where his colors go, without asking, who will fight a phantom foe in jungle and mountain range, without counting, and who will suffer and die in the midst of incredible hardship, without complaint, is still what he always has been, from Imperial Rome to sceptered Britain to democratic America. He is the stuff of which legions are made.
>
> His pride is in his colors and his regiment, his training hard and thorough and coldly realistic, to fit him for what he must face, and his obedience to his orders. As a legionary, he held the gates of civilization for the classical world; as a bluecoated horseman, he swept the Indians from the Plains; he has been called United States Marine. He does the jobs—the utterly necessary jobs—no militia is willing to do. His task is moral or immoral according to the orders that send him forth.[47]

This vision, whether alluring or not at this point, is all too familiar. For some a dream and for others a nightmare, it has undeniably come true.

47. Fehrenbach, *This Kind of War*, 658.

Legions, we know from history as well as from recent experience, belong to empires not democracies. And therein lies the problem.

> From the dawn of history wise men have seen that the perpetuation of free institutions depends on the power of self-defense. To be permanent, democratic political institutions must include a democratic system of military security.... A free state cannot continue to be democratic in peace and autocratic in war. Standing armies threaten government by the people, not because they consciously seek to pervert liberty but because they relieve the people themselves of the duty of self-defense. A people accustomed to let a special class defend them must sooner or later become unfit for liberty. An enduring government by the people must include an army of the people among its vital institutions. For this reason, the maintenance of a single professional soldier more than necessary threatens the very groundwork of free institutions.[48]

George Marshall, the first army general to be appointed to five-star rank and later secretary of state, in his final report as U.S. Army chief of staff to the secretary of war in the summer of 1945, referenced the "German" view that "an invincible offensive military force . . . could win any political argument" and commented that

> This is the doctrine Hitler carried to the verge of complete success. It is the doctrine of Japan. It is a criminal doctrine, and like other forms of crime, it has cropped up again and again since man began to live with his neighbors in communities and nations. There has long been an effort to outlaw war for exactly the same reason that man has outlawed murder. But the law prohibiting murder does not of itself prevent murder. It must be enforced. The enforcing power, however, must be maintained on a strictly democratic basis. There must not be a large standing army subject to the behest of a group of schemers. The citizen-soldier is the guarantee against such a misuse of power.[49]

Needless to say we have not heeded Marshall's words. As many would say, bent on empire, we have found legions more useful than a citizen army. Fixated on hegemony, America seems satisfied to be a superpower, *the* superpower, if nothing else, the nation with the biggest fist. Growing up in that clenched fist, we are, in Plato's words, being "trained insufficiently or amiss," and we pay a daily price for it. We are a nation of fear, not only

48. Palmer, *Statesmanship or War*, 74.
49. U.S. War Department General Staff, *Biennial Report*, 117.

at war with others but at war with ourselves. Peace is what we find in the privacy of our homes, if at all. But how would a return to a citizen army change any of this for the better?

For one thing, it just might put a brake on American military adventurism. Without a standing army capable of fighting several wars simultaneously, which is what is currently regarded as "readiness," we would be slower to embark on disaster. "As long as the tradition of the citizen-soldier remains moribund," writes West Point graduate and retired Army Colonel Andrew Bacevich, "reversing the militarization of U.S. foreign policy will be a pipe dream."[50]

More to the immediate point, perhaps, with universal conscription every citizen would have a more equal stake in the nation and would pay a fair and equal price for the security and advantages we all enjoy. Common service might serve to patch together our torn national fabric, rent by faction, fear, and contempt—particularly, if we were to take a further step to create what William James, in his last public utterance over a century ago, called "the moral equivalent of war."

A confirmed and outspoken pacifist, James considered it his "bounden duty" to "believe in [the possibility of] international rationality,"[51] by which he meant the capacity of human beings to settle their differences and to reach agreement without resorting to force. But he knew it would take more than this belief to make that happen. Pacifism, as he saw it envisioned and proposed by the antimilitarists of his day, offered no viable nor persuasive substitute for the unstinting idealism, discipline, courage, self-sacrifice, and fierce, intimate loyalty instilled and exemplified in military training and service. Instead, they offered a "pleasure economy," in which self-interest replaces selflessness, a society of each for himself. "I do not believe, wrote James, "that peace either ought to be or will be permanent on this globe, unless the states, pacifically organized, preserve some of the old elements of army-discipline."[52] To accomplish this, James proposed "instead of military conscription, a conscription of the whole youthful population to form for a certain number of years"[53] an "army" of a kind to address the needs of a peaceful nation, from building roads to hauling away the garbage.

---

50. Bacevich, "Whose Army?" 133.
51. James, "Moral Equivalent of War," 402.
52. Ibid., 407.
53. Ibid., 408.

> Such a conscription, with the state of public opinion that would have required it, and the many moral fruits it would bear, would preserve in the midst of a pacific civilization the manly virtues which the military party is so afraid of seeing disappear in peace. We should get toughness without callousness, authority with as little criminal cruelty as possible, and painful work done cheerily because the duty is temporary, and threatens not, as now, to degrade the whole remainder of one's life.[54]

We might well set loftier goals than James proposed for the tasks assigned to such an army of youth, but James' point is well made. Pacifism cannot be about selfishness and expect to preserve a nation, much less challenge it to greatness. On this point he was convinced that "the martial type of character can be bred without war":

> Strenuous honor and disinterestedness abound everywhere. Priests and medical men are in a fashion educated to it, and we should all feel some degree of its imperative if we were conscious of our work as an obligatory service to the state. We should be *owned*, as soldiers are by the army, and our pride would rise accordingly. We could be poor, then, without humiliation, as army officers now are. The only thing needed henceforward is to inflame the civic temper as past history has inflamed the military temper.[55]

Now, a century after these words were written, we would, of course, want to revise and add to James' list of those displaying in their civilian lives the selfless responsibility and commitment we expect and recognize in our armed servicemen and women. But in the end it comes to this: service is the soul of a country. Without it we are unable to go to war, and without it we will never be able to leave war behind us. "The soul of peacemaking," writes Daniel Berrigan, is "simply the will to give one's life."[56] War has never been possible unless men have been willing to kill each other and, while they're at it, possibly to be killed. We would be deluded, I believe, if we were to imagine that a future, unbroken peace will ever be brought about or preserved merely by an unwillingness to kill. Peacemakers, like warmakers, must be prepared to give up their lives—or as James would have it, at least several years of their lives—to the daunting but not impossible challenge of creating a moral alternative to war.

54. Ibid.
55. Ibid., 409.
56. Berrigan, *To Dwell in Peace*, 223.

Afterword

U PON COMPLETING *Killing from the Inside Out,* I did not know whether to lock myself in my house and weep, or to run screaming through the streets, "Repent! Repent!" Making war has apparently become as addictive to American political leaders as crack cocaine or heroin.

Over the last fifteen or so years I have gotten to know a substantial number of American military officers, as a "missionary" to the U.S. Armed Forces (sent by the psychologically and morally injured veterans I served as a V.A. psychiatrist)—a missionary on *prevention* of psychological and moral injury in military service. I have never yet met an officer who loves war. I expect that there must be some. Possibly they sheer off when they see me coming, so I haven't met them. Perhaps I have become too well known for them to say what they really think. However, at least one Marine officer, James N. Mattis, who was my direct boss for the *Commandant of the Marine Corps Trust Study* in 1999–2000, and treasured friend since then, has *never* short-changed me by less-than-complete candor.

Getting to know these officers—many Marines, many Army infantry and armor, hardly any Air Force, a few Navy—I have many times encountered a deep attachment to the Roman Catholic religious doctrine, known as Just War Doctrine, whether they were Roman Catholic or not. I forecast that the clarity of this book will make them squirm, because Just War Doctrine has become as American as apple pie. It spells out their patriotism of "For God and Country." For them, Just War Doctrine is inseparable from their understanding of the legal principle of civilian control of the Armed Forces, because there is no doubt in their minds that the "Sovereign" in the American polity is civilian. After all, didn't George Washington take off his military uniform when he became President? But I suspect the doctrine sits less comfortably with their understanding of the Commissioned Officer's Oath of Office under Section 3331, Title 5, United States Code, which is an oath to support and defend the Constitution, obedience to the President not mentioned.

Many are devout Christians, and just as devout American Soldiers, Marines, Sailors, Airmen. They will bridle at the stark flip-flop executed by Christian thought on war and military service—from comprehensively pacifistic before Emperor Constantine's conversion to Christianity to downright warlike after his conversion. This was no less the conversion of the Roman legions, an army in which Christians had been discouraged if not banned from serving, to an army *requiring* Christian baptism.

I do not come from the rigorous Roman Catholic education of my dear friend, Bob Meagher, whom I have known mainly as a classicist, not a Church historian or theologian. Only recently did I learn that he is the author of an important book on St. Augustine—it was Augustine and Ambrose who first formulated the Christian Just War Doctrine. I have reason to suppose that Protestant theologians will not hold their noses, having recently read *Saving Paradise,* by theologians Brock and Parker, which paints essentially the same picture of pre-/post-Constantine flip-flop on war, but in fuller scholarly detail.

I hope this book will be read widely within the U.S. Armed Forces, bearing up under the squirming it will cause, and benefiting from the clarity that it brings.

Jonathan Shay, MD, PhD

Author of *Achilles in Vietnam: Combat Trauma and the Undoing of Character* and *Odysseus in America: Combat Trauma and the Trials of Homecoming.* Performer, *CMC Trust Study, 1999–2000,* Chair of Ethics, Leadership, and Personnel Policy in the Office of the U.S. Army Deputy Chief of Staff for Personnel (G-1), 2004–2005; 2009 Omar Bradley Chair of Strategic Leadership, U.S. Army War College.

Bibliography

Abelard, Peter. *Ethical Writings: "Ethics" and "Dialogue between a Philosopher, a Jew, and a Christian"*. Translated by Peter Vincent Spade. Indianapolis: Hackett, 1995.

Alpert, Jon, and Ellen Goosenberg Kent. *Wartorn 1861–2010*. New York: HBO Documentary Films, 2011.

Ambrose. *On the Duties of the Clergy*. Translated by H. de Romestin et al. In vol. 10 of *The Nicene and Post-Nicene Fathers*, Series 2. Edited by Philip Schaff.

Anscombe, G. E. M. "War and Murder." In *Nuclear Weapons: A Catholic Response*, edited by Walter Stein, 43–62. London: Merlin, 1961. http://philosophyfaculty.ucsd.edu/faculty/rarneson/Anscombe.pdf.

Aristotle. *The Basic Works of Aristotle*. Edited by Richard McKeon. New York: Random House, 1966.

———. *Rhetoric*. Translated by W. Rhys Roberts. In *The Basic Works of Aristotle*, edited by Richard McKeon. New York: Random House, 1966.

Augustine. *The City of God*. Translated by Marcus Dods. In vol. 2 of *The Nicene and Post-Nicene Fathers*, Series 1. Edited by Philip Schaff.

———. *Confessions*. Translated by Henry Chadwick. Oxford: Oxford University Press, 1991.

———. *Expositions on the Book of Psalms*. Translated by A. Cleveland Coxe. In vol. 8 of *The Nicene and Post-Nicene Fathers*, Series 1. Edited by Philip Schaff.

———. *Letters*. Translated by J. G. Cunningham. In vol. 1 of *The Nicene and Post-Nicene Fathers*, Series 1. Edited by Philip Schaff.

———. *Letters*. Vol. 3. Translated by Wilfrid Parsons. Fathers of the Church 20. Washington, DC: Catholic University of America Press, 1953.

———. *On Free Will*. In *Earlier Writings*, selected and translated by John H. S. Burleigh, 102–217. Library of Christian Classics 6. Philadelphia: Westminster, 1953.

———. *Reply to Faustus the Manichaean*. Translated by Richard Stothert. In vol. 4 of *The Nicene and Post-Nicene Fathers*, Series 1. Edited by Philip Schaff.

———. *Ten Homilies on the First Epistle of John*. Translated by H. Browne. In vol. 7 of *The Nicene and Post-Nicene Fathers*, Series 1. Edited by Philip Schaff.

Bacevich, Andrew J. "Whose Army?" *Daedalus* 140 (2011) 122–34.

Basil. *The Letters*. Translated by Marcus Dods. In vol. 8 of *The Nicene and Post-Nicene Fathers*, Series 2. Edited by Philip Schaff.

Bibliography

Bede. *Bede's Ecclesiastical History of England.* Translated by A. M. Sellar. London: George Bell, 1907.

Bernard of Clairvaux. *In Praise of the New Knighthood.* Translated by M. Conrad Greenia. Collegeville, MN: Liturgical, 2000.

Berrigan, Daniel. *To Dwell in Peace: An Autobiography.* San Francisco: Harper & Row, 1987.

Bettenson, Henry, ed. *Documents of the Christian Church.* 2nd ed. Oxford: Oxford University Press, 1963.

Boudreau, Tyler. *Packing Inferno: The Unmaking of a Marine.* Port Townsend, WA: Feral House, 2008.

Brown, Peter. *The Body and Society: Men, Women, and Sexual Renunciation in Early Christianity.* New York: Columbia University Press, 1988.

Burn, A. R. "*Hic Breve Vivitur*: A Study of the Expectation of Life in the Roman Empire." *Past and Present* 4 (1953) 2–31.

Campenhausen, Hans von. *Tradition and Life in the Church: Essays and Lectures in Church History.* Translated by A. V. Littledale. Philadelphia: Fortress, 1968.

Camus, Albert. *Neither Victims nor Executioners.* Translated by Dwight Macdonald. Berkeley: World Without War Council, 1968.

———. *The Rebel.* Translated by Anthony Bower. New York: Vintage, 1956.

Clement of Alexandria. *Stromateis.* Translated by William Wilson. In vol. 2 of *The Ante-Nicene Fathers.* Edited by Alexander Roberts and James Donaldson.

Cowdrey, H. E. J. "Bishop Ermenfrid of Sion and the Penitential Ordinance following the Battle of Hastings." *Journal of Ecclesiastical History* 20 (1969) 225–42.

———. "The Genesis of the Crusades: The Springs of Western Ideas of Holy War." In *The Holy War,* edited by Thomas Patrick Murphy, 9–32. Columbus: Ohio State University Press, 1976.

Cyprian of Carthage. *Epistles.* Translated by Ernest Wallis. In vol. 5 of *The Ante-Nicene Fathers.* Edited by Alexander Roberts and James Donaldson.

———. *Treatises.* Translated by Ernest Wallace. In vol. 5 of *The Ante-Nicene Fathers.* Edited by Alexander Roberts and James Donaldson.

Davis, Henry. *Moral and Pastoral Theology: A Summary.* New York: Sheed & Ward, 1952.

Didascalia Apostolorum. Translated by R. Hugh Connolly. Oxford: Clarendon, 1929.

Dionysius of Alexandria. *The Canons of Dionysius.* Translated by F. C. Conybeare. In vol. 9 of *The Nicene and Post-Nicene Fathers,* Series 2. Edited by Philip Schaff.

Dodds, E. R. *The Greeks and the Irrational.* Berkeley: University of California Press, 1971.

Erasmus, Desiderius. *The Collected Works of Erasmus.* Vol. 27. Translated by Neil M. Cheshire and Michael Heath. Toronto: University of Toronto Press, 1986.

Eusebius. *Demonstration of the Gospel.* Translated by W. J. Ferrar. New York: Macmillan, 1920.

———. *The Life of Constantine.* Translated by Arthur C. McGiffert and Ernest C. Richardson. In vol. 1 of *The Nicene and Post-Nicene Fathers,* Series 2. Edited by Philip Schaff.

———. *Oration of Eusebius in Praise of Constantine.* Translated by Arthur C. McGiffert and Ernest C. Richardson. In vol. 1 of *The Nicene and Post-Nicene Fathers,* Series 2. Edited by Philip Schaff.

Fehrenbach, Theodore R. *This Kind of War: A Study in Unpreparedness.* New York: Macmillan, 1963.

Forde, Steven. "Hugo Grotius on Ethics and War." *The American Political Science Review* 92 (1998) 639–48.

French, Shannon. *The Code of the Warrior: Exploring Warrior Values Past and Present.* Lanham, MD: Rowman & Littlefield, 2003.

Freud, Sigmund. *Civilization and Its Discontents.* Translated and edited by James Strachey. New York: Norton, 1961.

———. *Reflections on War and Death.* Translated by A. A. Brill and Alfred B. Kuttner. New York: Moffat, Yard, 1918.

Frier, Bruce. "Roman Life Expectancy: Ulpian's Evidence." *Harvard Studies in Classical Philology* 86 (1982) 213–51.

Geneva Conventions. Introduction by Gary D. Solis, annotations by Fred L. Borch. New York: Kaplan, 2010.

Gilbertson, Ashley. "The Life and Lonely Death of Noah Pierce." *The Virginia Quarterly Review* (Fall 2008) 35–54. http://www.vqronline.org/vqr-portfolio/life-and-lonely-death-noah-pierce.

Girard, René. *Violence and the Sacred.* Translated by Patrick Gregory. Baltimore: Johns Hopkins University Press, 1972.

Glantz, Aaron, and Iraq Veterans Against the War. *Winter Soldier: Iraq and Afghanistan; Eyewitness Accounts of the Occupations.* Chicago: Haymarket, 2008.

Gray, J. Glenn. *The Warriors: Reflections on Men in Battle.* Lincoln, NE: Bison, 1998.

Grotius, Hugo. *De Iure Belli ac Pacis* [The Rights of War and Peace]. Translated by Francis W. Kelsey et al. Classics of International Law. Oxford: Clarendon, 1925.

Gutmann, Matthew, and Catherine Lutz, eds. *Breaking Ranks: Iraq Veterans Speak Out Against the War.* Berkeley: University of California Press, 2010.

Hippolytus. *The Apostolic Tradition of Hippolytus.* Translated by Burton Scott Easton. Hamden, CT: Archon, 1962.

Hobbes, Thomas. *Leviathan.* Baltimore: Pelican Classics, 1968.

Homer. *Iliad.* Translated by Stanley Lombardo. Indianapolis: Hackett, 1997.

James, William. "The Moral Equivalent of War." *Popular Science Monthly* 77 (1910) 400–410. http://en.wikisource.org/wiki/Popular_Science_Monthly/Volume_77/October_1910/The_Moral_Equivalent_of_War.

Jonas, Hans. "Change and Permanence: On the Possibility of Understanding History." *Social Research* 38 (1971) 498–528.

Junger, Sebastian. *War.* New York: Twelve, 2010.

Kirk, G. S., and J. E. Raven. *The Presocratic Philosophers.* Cambridge: Cambridge University Press, 1957.

Konstan, David. *Before Forgiveness: The Origins of a Moral Idea.* Cambridge: Cambridge University Press, 1962.

Kudo, Timothy. "I Killed People in Afghanistan. Was I Right or Wrong?" *Washington Post,* January 25, 2013. http://www.washingtonpost.com/opinions/i-killed-people-in-afghanistan-was-i-right-or-wrong/2013/01/25/c0b0d5a6-60ff-11e2-b05a-605528f6b712_story.html.

Kunz, Josef L. "Bellum Justum and Bellum Legale." *The American Journal of International Law* 45 (1951) 528–34.

Lactantius. *The Divine Institutes.* Translated by William Fletcher. In vol. 7 of *The Ante-Nicene Fathers.* Edited by Alexander Roberts and James Donaldson.

———. *The Epitome of the Divine Institutes.* Translated by William Fletcher. In vol. 7 of *The Ante-Nicene Fathers.* Edited by Alexander Roberts and James Donaldson.

Laffan, R. G. D., ed. *Select Documents of European History, 800–1492*. New York: Henry Holt, 1929.

Linn, Brian McAllister. "The U.S. Armed Forces' View of War." *Daedalus* 140 (2011) 33–44.

MacNair, Rachel M. *Perpetration-Induced Traumatic Stress: The Psychological Consequences of Killing*. Westport, CT: Praeger, 2002.

Mahedy, William P. *Out of the Night: The Spiritual Journey of Vietnam Vets*. New York: Ballantine, 1986.

Malraux, André. *Man's Fate*. Translated by Haakon M. Chevalier. New York: Modern Library, 1934.

Markus, R. A. "Two Conceptions of Political Authority: Augustine, *De Civitate Dei*, XIX.14–15, and Some Thirteenth-Century Interpretations." *Journal of Theological Studies* 16 (1965) 68–100.

Marlantes, Karl. *What It Is Like to Go to War*. New York: Atlantic Monthly Press, 2011.

Martens, G. F. de. *Précis du Droit des Gens de l'Europe* (1789). In *Compendium of the Law of Nations*. Translated by William Cobbett. London: Cobbett and Morgan, 1802.

Mattox, John Mark. *Saint Augustine and the Theory of Just War*. New York: Continuum, 2006.

McBride, William Leon. *The Development and Meaning of Twentieth-Century Existentialism*. Philadelphia: Taylor and Francis, 1997.

Meagher, Robert Emmet. *The Essential Euripides: Dancing in Dark Times*. Wauconda, IL: Bolchazy-Carducci, 2002.

———. *Herakles Gone Mad: Rethinking Heroism in an Age of Endless War*. Northampton, MA: Olive Branch, 2006.

Meyer, Kuno, ed. and trans. *Cáin Adamnáin: An Old Irish Treatise on the Law of Adamnan*. Oxford: Clarendon, 1905.

Morris, Errol. *The Fog of War: Eleven Lessons from the Life of Robert S. McNamara*. Documentary film transcript. http://www.errolmorris.com/film/fow_transcript.html.

Mullaney, Craig M. *The Unforgiving Minute: A Soldier's Education*. New York: Penguin, 2010.

Nagl, John A. "Let's Win the Wars We're In." *Joint Force Quarterly* 52 (1st Quarter 2009) 20–26.

Nussbaum, Arthur. "Just War—A Legal Concept?" *Michigan Law Review* 42 (1943) 453–79.

Obama, Barack. "Nobel Lecture." http://www.nobelprize.org/nobel_prizes/peace/laureates/2009/obama-lecture_en.html.

O'Brien, Tim. *The Things They Carried*. New York: Broadway, 1998.

O'Grady, Kathleen. "The Semantics of Taboo: Menstrual Prohibitions in the Hebrew Bible." In *Wholly Woman, Holy Blood: A Feminist Critique of Purity and Impurity*, edited by Kristin de Troyer et al., 1–28. Harrisburg, PA: Trinity, 2003.

Origen. *Against Celsus*. Translated by Frederick Crombie. In vol. 4 of *The Ante-Nicene Fathers*. Edited by Alexander Roberts and James Donaldson.

Palmer, John McAuley. *Statesmanship or War*. Garden City, NY: Doubleday, Page, 1927.

Parker, Robert. *Miasma: Pollution and Purification in Early Greek Religion*. Oxford: Clarendon, 1983.

Plato. *The Collected Dialogues of Plato, Including the Letters*. Edited by Edith Hamilton and Huntington Cairns. New York: Pantheon, 1961.

Prager, Dennis. "A Morally Confused Marine." *National Review*, February 5, 2013. http://www.nationalreview.com/articles/339804/morally-confused-marine-dennis-prager.

Roberts, Alexander, et al., eds. *The Ante-Nicene Fathers*. 10 vols. 1867–1885. Reprint, Grand Rapids: Eerdmans, 1989–1990. http://www.ccel.org/fathers.html.

Robinson, J. H. *Readings in European History*. Boston: Ginn, 1905.

Russell, Frederick H. *The Just War in the Middle Ages*. Cambridge: Cambridge University Press, 1977.

Sappho. *Sappho*. Translated by Mary Barnard. Berkeley: University of California Press, 1958.

Sassoon, Siegfried. *The War Poems of Siegfried Sassoon*. Seaside, OR: Merchant, 1919.

Schaff, Philip, et al., eds. *The Nicene and Post-Nicene Fathers*. Series 1. 14 vols. 1885. Reprint, Peabody, MA: Hendrickson, 1989. http://www.ccel.org/fathers.html.

———. *The Nicene and Post-Nicene Fathers*. Series 2. 14 vols. 1885. Reprint, Peabody, MA: Hendrickson, 1994. http://www.ccel.org/fathers.html.

Schroeder, H. J., ed. *Disciplinary Decrees of the General Councils: Text, Translation, and Commentary*. St. Louis: Herder, 1937.

Shalikashvili, John M. *Joint Vision 2010*. Washington, DC: Department of Defense, 2010. http://www.dtic.mil/jv2010/jv2010.pdf.

Shay, Jonathan. *Achilles in Vietnam: Combat Trauma and the Undoing of Character*. New York: Athenaeum, 1994.

———. *Odysseus in America: Combat Trauma and the Trials of Homecoming*. New York: Scribner, 2002.

Socrates Scholasticus. *Ecclesiastical History*. Translated by A. C. Zenos. In vol. 2 of *The Nicene and Post-Nicene Fathers*, Series 2. Edited by Philip Schaff.

Sophocles. *Oedipus at Colonus*. Translated by Robert Fitzgerald. In *Sophocles*, edited by David Grene and Richmond Lattimore, 2:77–155. Chicago: University of Chicago Press, 1957.

———. *Oedipus the King*. Translated by David Grene. In *Sophocles*, edited by David Grene and Richmond Lattimore, 1:9–76. Chicago: University of Chicago Press, 1954.

———. *Philoctetes*. Translated by David Grene. In *Sophocles*, edited by David Grene and Richmond Lattimore, 2:194–254. Chicago: University of Chicago Press, 1957.

Swift, Louis J. *The Early Fathers on War and Military Service*. Wilmington, DE: Michael Glazier, 1983.

Tertullian. *Apology*. Translated by S. Thelwall. In vol. 3 of *The Ante-Nicene Fathers*. Edited by Alexander Roberts and James Donaldson.

———. *The Chaplet*. Translated by S. Thelwall. In vol. 3 of *The Ante-Nicene Fathers*. Edited by Alexander Roberts and James Donaldson.

———. *On Exhortation to Chastity*. Translated by S. Thelwall. In vol. 3 of *The Ante-Nicene Fathers*. Edited by Alexander Roberts and James Donaldson.

———. *On Idolatry*. Translated by S. Thelwall. In vol. 3 of *The Ante-Nicene Fathers*. Edited by Alexander Roberts and James Donaldson.

Theodoret. *Ecclesiastical History*. Translated by Blomfield Jackson. In vol. 3 of *The Nicene and Post-Nicene Fathers*, Series 2. Edited by Philip Schaff.

Thomas, Aquinas. *Summa Theologica*. Translated by Fathers of the English Dominican Province. London: Burns, Oates & Washbourne, 1920. http://www.newadvent.org/summa/index.html.

Thucydides. *History of the Peloponnesian War*. Translated by Rex Warner. New York: Penguin, 1954.

Bibliography

Turner, Brian. *Here, Bullet*. Farmington, ME: Alice James, 2005.

United States War Department General Staff. *Biennial Report of the Chief of Staff of the United States Army, July 1, 1943, to June 30, 1945, to the Secretary of War*. Washington, DC: Infantry Journal Press, 1945.

Upton-Ward, J. M. *The Rule of the Templars*. Rochester, NY: Boydell, 2002.

Van Creveld, Martin. *The Transformation of War*. New York: Free Press, 1991.

Vattel, Emer de. *The Law of Nations, or Principles of the Law of Nature Applied to the Conduct and Affairs of Nations and Sovereigns*. Edited by Joseph Chitty. Philadelphia: T. & J. W. Johnson, 1883.

Verkamp, Bernard J. *The Moral Treatment of Returning Warriors in Early Medieval and Modern Times*. Scranton, PA: University of Scranton, 2006.

Vermeule, Emily. *Aspects of Death in Early Greek Art and Poetry*. Berkeley: University of California Press, 1979.

Victoria, Franciscus de. *De Indis et De Iure Belli Relectiones* [On the Amerindians and On the Law of War]. Translated by Herbert Francis Wright. Classics of International Law. Oxford: Clarendon, 1925.

Weil, Simone. *The Iliad, or The Poem of Force*. Translated by Mary McCarthy. Wallingford, PA: Pendle Hill, 1956.

Weingarten, Gene. "Fatal Distraction: Forgetting a Child in the Backseat of a Car Is a Horrifying Mistake. Is It a Crime?" *Washington Post*, March 8, 2011. http://www.washingtonpost.com/wp-dyn/content/article/2009/02/27/AR2009022701549.html.

White, Josh. "Prince William Mother Charged with Felony Murder in Toddler's Hot-Van Death." *Washington Post*, July 5, 2011. http://www.washingtonpost.com/local/prince-william-mother-who-left-toddler-in-van-charged-with-felony-murder/2011/07/05/gHQA7A5pzH_story.html.

Williams, John. "Writing Differently about War, but Drawing from the Same Rich Vein." *New York Times*, November 13, 2012. http://nytimes.com/2012/11/13/books/kevin-powers-and-ben-fountain-national-book-award-nominees.html?

Woolf, Virginia. *Mrs. Dalloway*. http://ebooks.adelaide.edu.au/w/woolf/virginia/w91md/.

Zoroya, Greg. "Military Leaders Must Help Stem Suicides, Panetta Says." *USA Today*, September 16, 2012. http://usatoday30.usatoday.com/news/nation/story/2012/09/16/military-leaders-must-help-stem-suicides-panetta-says/57789420/1.

Index

www.ingramcontent.com/pod-product-compliance
Lightning Source LLC
Chambersburg PA
CBHW030845270326
41928CB00007B/1231